HANDBOOK OF GLAUCOMA

Dedication

To Noemi
Augusto Azuara-Blanco

Ana Paula, Bruno and Otavio
Vital P Costa

Karen
Richard P Wilson

HANDBOOK OF GLAUCOMA

Augusto Azuara-Blanco MD, PhD
Consultant Ophthalmic Surgeon
Aberdeen Royal Infirmary
Clinical Senior Lecturer
University of Aberdeen
Aberdeen
UK

Vital P Costa MD
Director, Glaucoma Service
University of Campinas, Brazil
Associate Professor of Ophthalmology (Post-Graduation),
University of Campinas
Associate Professor of Ophthalmology (Post-Graduation)
University of San Paolo, Brazil

Richard P Wilson MD
Attending Surgeon, Glaucoma Service
Wills Eye Hospital
Professor of Ophthalmology
Jefferson Medical College
Thomas Jefferson University
Philadelphia PA
USA

MARTIN DUNITZ

© 2002 Martin Dunitz Ltd, a member of the Taylor & Francis Group

First published in the United Kingdom in 2002
by Martin Dunitz Ltd, The Livery House, 7–9 Pratt Street,
0AE

Tel.:   +44 (0) 20 74822202
Fax.:   +44 (0) 20 72670159
E-mail: info@dunitz.co.uk
Website: http://www.dunitz.co.uk

A CIP record for this book is available from the British Library.

ISBN 1-841840-43-2

Distributed in the USA by
Fulfilment Center
Taylor & Francis
7625 Empire Drive
Florence, KY 41042
USA
Toll free tel: 1-800-634-7064
E-mail: cserve@routledge_ny.com

Distributed in Canada by
Taylor & Francis
74 Rolark Drive
Scarborough
Ontario M1R G2
Canada
Toll free tel: 1-877-226-2237
E-mail: tal_fran@istar.com

Distributed in the rest of the world by
ITPS Limited
Cheriton House
North Way
Andover
Hampshire SP10 5BE
UK
Tel: +44 (0)1264 332424
E-mail: reception@itps.co.uk

Composition by Scribe Design, Gillingham, Kent
Printed and bound in Singapore by Kyodo Printing Co (S'pore) Pte Ltd

CONTENTS

III Treatment

CONTRIBUTORS

Augusto Azuara-Blanco MD, PhD
Consultant Ophthalmic Surgeon
Aberdeen Royal Infirmary
Clinical Senior Lecturer
University of Aberdeen
Aberdeen AB25 2ZN
UK

Vital P Costa MD
Director, Glaucoma Service
University of Campinas, Brazil
Associate Professor of Ophthalmology (Post-Graduation),
University of Campinas
Associate Professor of Ophthalmology (Post-Graduation)
University of San Paolo
Sao Paolo 01234-000
Brazil

Sai B Gandham MD
Assistant Professor and Director, Glaucoma Unit
The Albany Medical College
Lions Eye Institute
Albany NY 12208
USA

Martha Motuz Leen MD
Clinical Assistant Professor
Department of Ophthalmology
University of Washington;
Pacific EyeCare
Bremerton
Poulsbo WA 98370
USA

Mark R Lesk MD
Clinical Assistant Professor
Department of Ophthalmology
School of Medicine
University of Montreal
Montreal
Quebec
Canada

Jeffrey M Liebmann MD
Professor of Clinical Ophthalmology
New York Medical College
Associate Director, Glaucoma Service
The New York Eye and Ear Infirmary
New York NY 10003
USA

Jeannette G Maresco MD
Lions Eye Institute
Albany NY 12208
USA

André Mermoud MD, PD
Head, Glaucoma Unit
Hôpital Ophtalmique Jules Gonin
University of Lausanne
Lausanne
Switzerland

Robert Ritch MD
Professor Clinical Ophthalmology
New York Medical College
Chief, Glaucoma Service
The New York Eye and Ear Infirmary
New York NY 10003
USA

Tarek Shaarawy MD
Head, Glaucoma Unit
Memorial Research Institute of Ophthalmology
Giza
Egypt

Celso Tello MD
Clinical Assistant Professor of Ophthalmology
New York Medical College
Glaucoma Service
The New York Eye and Ear Infirmary
New York NY 10003
USA

Richard P Wilson MD
Attending Eye Surgeon, Glaucoma Service
Wills Eye Hospital
Professor of Ophthalmology
Jefferson Medical College
Thomas Jefferson University
Philadelphia PA 19107
USA

PREFACE

The goal of *Handbook of Glaucoma* is to provide practical clinical information about the management of glaucoma in a concise text. The book is written for both practising ophthalmologists and ophthalmologists in training. We have tried to integrate the essential clinical manifestations, diagnostic technologies and therapeutic modalities of this group of diseases. We have also included the important recent developments in the pathogenesis and management of the different types of glaucoma; for example, practical guidelines for the interpretation of standard and new visual field tests (SITA algorithm) are provided. A large number of drugs have been recently introduced for the treatment of glaucoma and the clinical use of drugs for glaucoma therapy has greatly evolved, adapting with the advent of each new drug. The surgical outcome of guarded filtration surgery continues to improve with the use of antifibrotic agents, but an impeccable surgical technique is needed to avoid short- and long-term complications. A separate chapter has been dedicated to non-penetrating glaucoma surgery. We have used more than 200 illustrations and numerous tables to provide a natural and easily understandable flow of information.

Augusto Azuara-Blanco
Vital P Costa
Richard P Wilson

ACKNOWLEDGEMENTS

We are indebted to the contributors to this book for giving so generously their time and work. They are all recognized for their clinical and research expertise in their subject, and have authored excellent chapters: Drs Celso Tello, Jeffrey M Liebmann, and Robert Ritch (Examination of the anterior chamber angle); Dr Martha M Leen (Glaucoma laser procedures); Drs Tarek Shaarawy and André Mermoud (Non-penetrating glaucoma surgery); Drs Sai B Gandham and Jeannette G Maresco (Anatomy, physiology, and pathophysiology), and Dr Mark Lesk (The intraocular pressure in glaucoma). We are also extremely grateful to Alan Burgess, our commissioning editor at Martin Dunitz Ltd, for his help, patience, and advice, and to Charlotte Mossop for her expert editorial assistance.

SECTION I

BACKGROUND TO ANATOMY AND PATHOPHYSIOLOGY, CLASSIFICATION AND EXAMINATION

1. ANATOMY, PHYSIOLOGY AND PATHOPHYSIOLOGY

Jeannette G Maresco and Sai Gandham

The ciliary body

Anatomy and vascularization

The ciliary body, along with the iris and choroid, form the uveal tract. The ciliary body extends posteriorly 6 mm from the scleral spur to the ora serrata. It consists of ciliary muscle, ciliary processes (pars plicata), and the pars plana, the posterior 4 mm of the ciliary body.

Ciliary muscle

There are three ciliary muscle layers distinguished by the direction of their muscle fibers: the longitudinal, circular and radial layers. The longitudinal fibers are on the outermost part of the ciliary body, attaching it to the scleral spur and corneoscleral trabecular meshwork anteriorly. Posteriorly, a portion of the muscle inserts into the suprachoroidal lamina at the ora serrata. The inner circular fibers are located in the anterior portions of the ciliary body and run parallel to the limbus. The longitudinal and circular fibers are connected to each other via the radial layer.

Ciliary processes (pars plicata)

Lying internal to the ciliary muscle, the ciliary processes project radially into the posterior chamber. The anterior portion of the pars plicata is located about 1.5 to 2 mm posterior to the corneoscleral limbus. There are around 70 major ciliary processes that are about 2 mm in length, 0.5 mm in width, and 1 mm in height, and have an irregular surface. Smaller minor ciliary processes lie between major ones. Each major process is comprised of an inner capillary core, a surrounding loose stroma, and a double-layered epithelium, made up of an outer pigmented and inner non-pigmented layer of cells (Figure 1.1). These cells are joined apex to apex, with the pigmented layer facing the stroma and the non-pigmented layer lining the posterior chamber. The ciliary epithelial cells are interconnected by specialized intercellular junctions that control the passage of water, ions and macromolecules into the aqueous humor. Desmosomes and gap junctions lie between adjacent cells maintaining a small space between them (i.e. intercellular cleft). Near their apical surfaces, non-pigmented cells are joined by zonulae occludens, or tight junctions, that occlude the intercellular cleft and constitute the

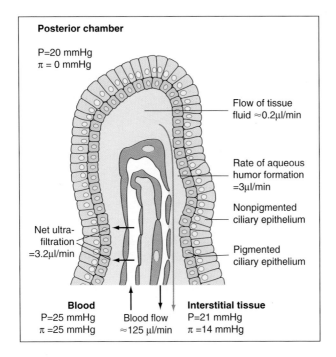

Figure 1.1 Ciliary process epithelium and production of aqueous humor. The ciliary process consists of a core containing capillaries and interstitial tissue surrounded by two epithelial layers oriented apex to apex. The inner layer consists of non-pigmented ciliary epithelial cells connected to each other by tight junctions and desmosomes. The outer layer consists of pigmented ciliary epithelial cells connected to each other by gap junctions. Plasma filtrate enters the interstitial space through capillary fenestrations (ultrafiltration). The non-pigmented ciliary epithelium acts as a barrier for the plasma proteins. The high protein concentration in the tissue fluid causes a high oncotic pressure. The hydrostatic pressure (P) and osmotic pressure (π) of the blood, interstitial tissue and posterior chamber are listed (for the rabbit). The effect of hydrostatic and oncotic pressure differences across the ciliary epithelium is a pressure of about 13 mmHg, tending to move water into the processes from the posterior chamber. Active transport across the ciliary epithelial layers is required to secrete fluid into the posterior chamber. Reproduced with permission from Toris CB, Yablonski ME, Tamesis R. Aqueous humor dynamics. In: Choplin NT, Lundy DC, eds. Atlas of Glaucoma. London; Martin Dunitz, 1998.

blood–aqueous barrier of the ciliary body. The tight junctions allow diffusion of water and small molecules into the posterior chamber, while maintaining the osmotic and electrical gradients across the ciliary epithelium that are required for the final, active step in aqueous humor production.

4

Ciliary body vascularization

The ciliary body receives blood from two sources: the anterior ciliary arteries and the long posterior ciliary arteries, with numerous branches that anastomose with each other. At the limbus, several branches from each anterior ciliary artery turn inward, perforating the limbal sclera to enter the capillary bed of the ciliary muscle. These branches arborize within the ciliary muscle and interconnect with each other and with branches from the nasal and temporal long posterior ciliary arteries. These interconnections form a vascular ring—the intramuscular circle. Other branches from the intramuscular circle pass anterior to the root of the iris, where they bend and branch at right angles to form the major arterial circle, which lies tangential to the limbus.

The ciliary processes have a highly vascularized core. They receive their arterial supply from two types of arterioles—anterior and posterior—that emanate from the major arterial circle. The tips of the ciliary processes are supplied by anterior branches, whereas the posterior branches deliver blood to the basal region

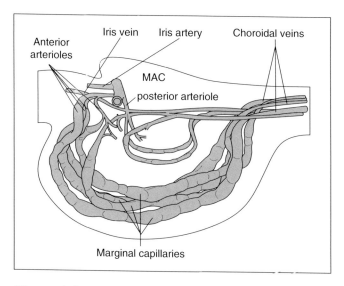

Figure 1.2 Ciliary processes vasculature. One ciliary process of a monkey is shown in lateral view. The vasculature consists of a complex anastomotic system supplied by anterior and posterior arterioles radiating from the major arterial circle (MAC). The anterior arterioles supply the anterior aspect of the process and drain posteriorly into the choroidal veins. The posterior arterioles provide posteriorly-draining capillaries confined to the base of the process. Reproduced with permission from Toris CB, Yablonski ME, Tamesis R. Aqueous humor dynamics. In: Choplin NT, Lundy DC, eds. Atlas of Glaucoma. London; Martin Dunitz, 1998.

of the ciliary processes. The anterior arterioles, as they enter the processes, rapidly dilate into large, irregular, vein-like fenestrated capillaries (Figure 1.2). The capillaries allow for the exchange of solutes between the blood and the stroma.

Production of aqueous humor

The primary function of the ciliary processes is to produce aqueous humor. The abundant blood vessels in the stroma of the ciliary processes are fenestrated, providing adequate fluid and ions for the production of aqueous humor. Such materials pass between the pigmented epithelial cells and accumulate in the intercellular cleft behind the tight junctions that join the non-pigmented cells. Next, an active transport of ions out of the non-pigmented epithelial cell establishes an osmotic gradient in the intercellular spaces of the ciliary epithe-

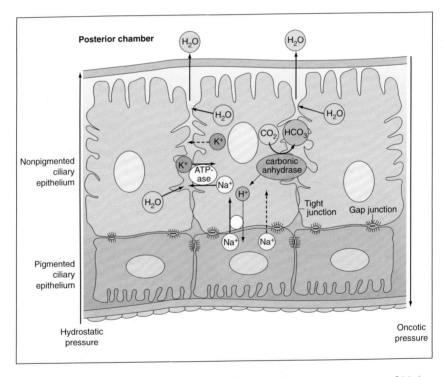

Figure 1.3 Active transport of aqueous humor. The active transport of Na^+ across the NPE is the key process in aqueous humor formation. Active transport of HCO_3^- and Cl^- may also play a role. Reproduced with permission from Toris CB, Yablonski ME, Tamesis R. Aqueous humor dynamics. In: Choplin NT, Lundy DC, eds. Atlas of Glaucoma. London; Martin Dunitz, 1998.

lium (Figure 1.3). Finally, water moves into the posterior chamber along the osmotic gradient. The posterior chamber aqueous humor is modified by diffusion of molecules into or out of the surrounding tissue. Normal rate of aqueous production is 2–2.5 microliters per minute. There is a circadian fluctuation in aqueous production, which is lowest during sleep. Aqueous production is also affected by age, decreasing by 2% per decade.

Functions of the aqueous humor

1 Aqueous flow helps to maintain the shape of the globe, which is a necessity for the structural integrity and optical function of the eye. It is contained by the posterior and the anterior chamber and has a volume of about 200 microliters.
2 Aqueous supplies substrates (e.g. oxygen, glucose, aminoacids) to cornea, lens and trabecular meshwork. Metabolic wastes (carbon dioxide, lactic acid) are removed from the anterior chamber.
3 Aqueous humor facilitates cellular and humoral immune responses under adverse conditions such as inflammation and infection.

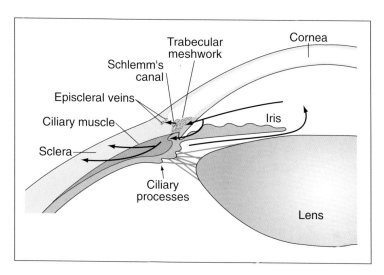

Figure 1.4 Circulation and drainage of aqueous humor. Aqueous humor is secreted by the ciliary processes into the posterior chamber. It circulates between the lens and the iris through the pupil into the anterior chamber (long, curved arrow). It drains from the anterior chamber by passive bulk via two pathways, trabecular outflow (to Schlemm's canal and episcleral veins) and uveoscleral outflow (into tissue spaces of the ciliary muscle, suprachoroidal space and through sclera). Reproduced with permission from Toris CB, Yablonski ME, Tamesis R. Aqueous humor dynamics. In: Choplin NT, Lundy DC, eds. Atlas of Glaucoma. London; Martin Dunitz, 1998.

Aqueous humor outflow

The conventional outflow pathway is pressure-dependent and represents 85–90% of the total outflow in adults. Moving from the anterior chamber outward, the aqueous travels through the trabecular meshwork and into Schlemm's canal (Figure 1.4). From Schlemm's canal, the aqueous enters the collector channels and flows through aqueous veins to the episcleral or conjunc-

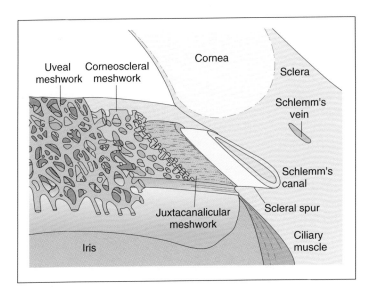

Figure 1.5 Three layers of the trabecular meshwork. Aqueous humor first passes through the inner layer of the uveal meshwork. This layer is a forward extension of the ciliary muscle. It consists of flattened sheets, which branch and interconnect in multiple planes that do not offer any significant resistance to aqueous drainage. The middle layer, or the corneoscleral meshwork, includes several perforated sheets of connective tissue extending between the scleral spur and Schwalbe's line. The sheets are connected to each other by tissue strands and endothelial cells. The openings are very small, providing resistance to the flow of aqueous. The outer layer, or the juxtacanalicular meshwork, lies adjacent to the inner wall of Schlemm's canal. It contains collagen, glycosaminoglycans and glycoproteins, fibroblasts, and endothelial-like juxtacanalicular cells. It also contains elastic fibers that may provide support for the inner wall of Schlemm's canal. This meshwork contains very narrow, irregular openings providing high resistance to fluid drainage. Reproduced with permission from Toris CB, Yablonski ME, Tamesis R. Aqueous humor dynamics. In: Choplin NT, Lundy DC, eds. Atlas of Glaucoma. London; Martin Dunitz, 1998.

tival veins. From there, it proceeds through the anterior ciliary and superior ophthalmic veins to the cavernous sinus.

Non-conventional uveoscleral outflow accounts for the remaining 10–15% of the aqueous outflow in adults. Via this pressure independent pathway, the aqueous humor travels through the ciliary body face and iris root into the suprachoroidal space and out through the sclera into the orbital tissues. The younger the individual, the greater the proportion of aqueous exiting the eye by means of uveoscleral outflow. In children, 40–50% of outflow is through this non-conventional pathway.

The trabecular meshwork

Functionally, the scleral spur, ciliary muscle, trabecular meshwork and Schlemm's canal work as a unit to comprise the conventional aqueous outflow pathway. The trabecular meshwork lies in the anterior chamber angle, between the scleral spur posteriorly and Schwalbe's line anteriorly. In cross-section, the trabecular meshwork has a triangular shape, its apex at Schwalbe's line, and the base formed by the scleral spur and the inner fibers of the ciliary muscle, the inner wall facing the anterior chamber, and the outer wall comprising the inner wall of the Schlemm's canal.

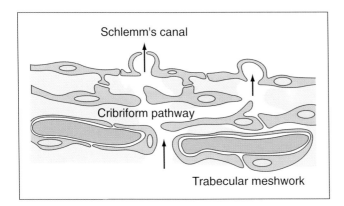

Figure 1.6 Inner wall of Schlemm's canal and the juxtacanalicular meshwork. The inner wall of Schlemm's canal contains a monolayer of spindle-shaped endothelial cells interconnected by tight junctions. Fluid may move through this area in transcellular channels. Only a few channels appear to open at a time, providing the major resistance to trabecular outflow. One channel is drawn as a vacuole and one is shown opened to Schlemm's canal. The arrows indicate the direction of fluid flow. Reproduced with permission from Toris CB, Yablonski ME, Tamesis R. Aqueous humor dynamics. In: Choplin NT, Lundy DC, eds. Atlas of Glaucoma. London; Martin Dunitz, 1998.

The trabecular meshwork consists of three components: the inner uveal meshwork, the central corneoscleral meshwork, and the outer juxta-canalicular tissue (Figure 1.5). The inner layers do not provide resistance to aqueous outflow. The juxtacanalicular tissue offers the main resistance to aqueous outflow. It consists of a layer of connective tissue lined on either side by endothelium: the outer layer of endothelium is part of Schlemm's canal and the inner layer is continuous with the trabecular endothelium (Figure 1.6). Cellular depopulation and accumulation of extracellular material, appearing as 'plaques' in electronmicroscopy sections, are associated with aging but are accelerated and exaggerated in open-angle glaucoma.

The connective tissue has elastic fibers that are connected with tendons of the ciliary muscle. Contraction of the ciliary muscle may increase spaces between the plates of the meshwork and reduce resistance to conventional outflow.

The optic nerve

The optic nerve is a cylindrical structure about 50 mm long situated between the retina and the chiasm, and can be divided topographically into four parts: 1) intraocular, or optic nerve head; 2) intraorbital, situated between the globe and the optic canal (25 mm long); 3) intracanalicular, localized within the optic canal (4–20 mm long); and 4) intracranial (10 mm long), situated between the optic canal and the chiasm.

The optic nerve is composed primarily of neural fibers (the retinal ganglion cell axons), glial cells, extracellular matrix supportive tissue, and vascular elements. The neural component of the optic nerve is composed of about 1.2–1.5 million axons. The axons originate in the neuron cell bodies located in the ganglion cell layer of the retina, and form the retinal nerve fiber layer to synapse in the lateral geniculate body. The axons of the ganglion cells nasal to the optic disc run directly toward the optic nerve head, similarly to the axons originated in the macular area, which form the spindle-shaped papillo-macular bundle. The axons coming from ganglion cells situated in the temporal fundus describe an arcuate course around the fovea and run toward the superior or inferior poles of the optic disc. These are the fibers most susceptible to early glaucomatous damage. The nerve-fiber layer is thickest at the vertical optic disc poles and thinnest at the temporal and nasal optic disc borders.

The ganglion cell axons are retinotopically organized as they travel into the optic nerve. Axons from the peripheral retina travel in the peripheral position of the retinal nerve fiber layer and optic nerve. Axons from the central part of the retina take a more superficial path in the nerve fiber layer and follow the innermost central part within the optic nerve (Figure 1.7).

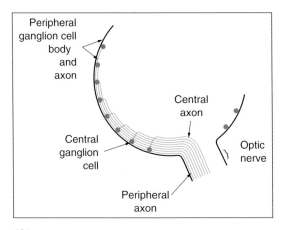

(A)

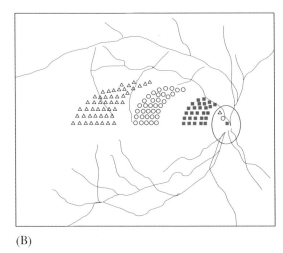

(B)

Figure 1.7 Retinotopic organization of the ganglion cell axons. (A) The retinotopic organization of the ganglion cell axons as they enter the optic nerve. Note that axons from peripheral retinal ganglion cells occupy a more peripheral position in the optic nerve. Axons from retinal areas closer to the disc are located more centrally in the nerve. (B) A frontal view of the distribution pattern of axons as shown in (A). The same retina-optic nerve correspondence of fibers is represented. Reproduced with permission from Gamero GE, Fechtner RD. The optic nerve in glaucoma. In: Choplin NT, Lundy DC, eds. Atlas of Glaucoma. London; Martin Dunitz, 1998.

There are two major types of retinal ganglion cells: the parvocellular (P) and magnocellular (M) cells. P cells are the most abundant and have smaller axon diameters, smaller receptive fields, and slower conduction velocities. P cells are sensitive to color and form (visual acuity), and synapse at the parvocellular layer in the lateral geniculate body. M cells are sensitive to changes in luminance in a dim environment and to moving targets, and allow temporal resolution. They synapse at the magnocellular layer in the lateral geniculate body. Some authors have proposed that there is preferential damage of M cells in early glaucoma. This possibility has stimulated the development of new methods to test the function of M cells (e.g. frequency doubling technology, motion perimetry, flicker perimetry). Further evidence is needed to confirm this hypothesis.

Anatomy of the optic nerve head

The optic nerve head, also known as optic disc or papilla, is delineated by the peripapillary scleral ring of Elschnig, a white band that separates the optic nerve head from the peripapillary retina. The optic nerve head is divided into four regions: the superficial nerve fiber layer, and the prelaminar, laminar, and retrolaminar areas (Figure 1.8).

(A) The superficial nerve fiber layer is continuous with the nerve fiber layer of the retina and is primarily composed of axons. The inner limiting membrane separates the vitreous from the nerve fiber layer. Over the optic nerve head cup, this layer thickens and is referred to as the central meniscus of Kuhnt.

(B) The prelaminar area, also known as the choroidal part, consists of nerve fiber bundles and astroglia forming tube-like sheaths around each bundle.

(C) The laminar or scleral portion of the optic disc includes a modification of the sclera called lamina cribrosa. The lamina cribrosa is bent slightly backward and comprises eight to 12 sheets of connective and elastic tissue. Each sheet has 500–600 irregularly disposed pores, which are aligned to form straight line channels through the lamina cribrosa. The fenestrations contain bundles of retinal nerve fibers, and are larger at the superior and inferior poles. The larger pores have thinner connective tissue and may be more vulnerable to damage. The main function of the lamina cribrosa is to

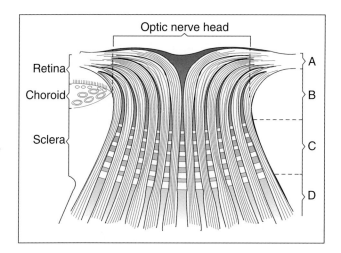

Figure 1.8 Schematic subdivision of the optic nerve head in four portions: A, Nerve fiber layer; B, Prelaminar; C, Laminar; D, Retrolaminar. Reproduced with permission from Gamero GE, Fechtner RD. The optic nerve in glaucoma. In: Choplin NT, Lundy DC, eds. Atlas of Glaucoma. London; Martin Dunitz, 1998.

give passage to the ganglion cell axons and the retinal blood vessels, while preserving intraocular pressure (IOP) against a gradient between the intraocular and extraocular spaces.

(D) The most posterior layer, the retrolaminar portion, is composed of myelinated fibers and is circumscribed by the leptomeninges of the central nervous system.

The optic nerve head is slightly vertically oval, with the vertical diameter being about 9% larger than the horizontal one. Morphometric studies have shown that its area varies between 0.86 and 5.86 mm^2, with a mean of 2.70 mm^2. In highly hyperopic eyes, the optic disc area tends to be smaller, whereas highly myopic eyes are associated with large optic discs.

When viewed stereoscopically, the neural component of the nerve head has an orange-pink tint. The neuroretinal rim represents the main focus of the optic disc evaluation in glaucoma. It is significantly broader in the inferior pole, and becomes progressively narrower at the superior, nasal, and finally the temporal disc region (ISN'T rule). Because the fibers change direction abruptly, bending centrifugally, a central concavity or 'cup' is created, the base of which appears more yellow-white because of the underlying collagenous fibers of the lamina cribrosa. The cups are horizontally oval, with the horizontal diameter being about 8% longer than the vertical diameter. The size and depth of the cup is highly variable, and depends on the size of the optic discs. This leads to important clinical guidelines: large discs may be associated with physiologically large

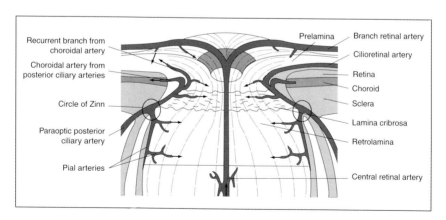

Figure 1.9 The arterial vasculature of the optic nerve head. Note the extensive contribution of the short posterior ciliary arteries as well as the intraneural branches from the central retinal artery in the retrolaminar region. Reproduced with permission from Gamero GE, Fechtner RD. The optic nerve in glaucoma. In: Choplin NT, Lundy DC, eds. Atlas of Glaucoma. London; Martin Dunitz, 1998.

cups, which resemble glaucomatous damage. On the other hand, apparently normal cups in small discs may already be a sign of glaucomatous damage.

Optic nerve head vascularization

The main arterial supply of the optic nerve derives from the short posterior ciliary arteries (Figure 1.9). However, some variations in different parts of the optic nerve head should be noted.

(A) The superficial nerve fiber layer receives blood from retinal arterioles branching from the central retinal artery. Capillaries in this layer are continuous with the retinal capillaries.

(B) The prelaminar region is supplied by direct branches from the short posterior ciliary arteries and by centripetal branches of the circle of Zinn-Haller, when it is present. The circle of Zinn-Haller is a terminal confluence of short posterior ciliary arteries and is variable in extent from being absent to quite prominent. In eyes with a well developed circle of Zinn-Haller, fine arterial branches supply both the prelaminar and laminar regions.

(C) The laminar region has a rich capillary plexus that is supplied by branches of the short posterior ciliary arteries or from the circle of Zinn-Haller, similar to the prelaminar region. There is no anastomosis between the capillaries of the prelaminar and laminar optic nerve and the choriocapillaries.

(D) The retrolaminar region is supplied by branches of the short posterior ciliary arteries and pial arterial vessels. The pial arteries originate from the central retinal artery before it pierces the retrobulbar optic nerve, and from branches of the short posterior ciliary arteries more anteriorly. The central retinal vein drains almost all four layers.

The blood vessels supplying the optic nerve head have tight junctions, nonfenestrated endothelium, and abundant pericytes that form the nerve-blood barrier. The vascular perfusion pressure of the optic nerve is defined as the difference between the mean local arterial pressure and the IOP. The arteries supplying blood to the optic nerve head can autoregulate, maintaining adequate blood flow despite variations in perfusion pressure. Optic nerve damage may occur when the perfusion pressure is insufficient to provide adequate blood flow to the nerve and when autoregulation mechanisms are impaired.

Pathophysiology of optic nerve damage in glaucoma

Obstruction of axoplasmic flow at the optic nerve head is probably involved in the pathogenesis of glaucomatous optic atrophy. However, it is still not clear whether mechanical and/or vascular factors primarily cause this damage and other alterations are also important in the ultimate loss of axons.

The mechanical and direct role of IOP in glaucoma is supported by cases with unilateral secondary glaucoma, experimentally induced glaucoma, and by the observation of the effects of IOP-lowering medications in patients with glaucoma. Eyes with extremely high IOP always develop cupping. According to the 'mechanical theory,' direct compression of axons associated with the deformation of the pores and channels of the lamina cribrosa would disrupt axoplasmic flow and lead to death of the ganglion cell. Electronmicroscopy has shown axonal transport blockage within a few hours of modest pressure increase. The larger laminar pore size and consequently the relative lack of connective tissue support in the superior and inferior regions of the lamina cribrosa could contribute to preferential damage of optic nerve axons in these regions compared with nasal and temporal regions of the lamina. However, not all cases with moderately increased IOP develop optic atrophy. In addition, cupping can occur without increased IOP. Ischemia may be the predominant pathogenetic factor in those glaucomas that occur with IOPs in the normal range. Impaired autoregulation in the arteries supplying the optic nerve head may compromise its perfusion, leading to ischemia and neural damage.

Mechanisms of cell death as they apply to the optic nerve are also under investigation. In glaucoma, retinal ganglion cells die by apoptosis, a genetically programmed process of cell death characterized histologically by chromatin condensation and intracellular fragmentation. It is known that when an axon dies, it releases excitatory neurotransmitters such as glutamate into the extracellular environment, which may trigger death of neighboring cells by apoptosis. An excessive release of glutamate in the retina may be associated with neuron cell death in glaucoma.

As the mechanisms leading to glaucoma become elucidated, new therapies may be developed to protect the optic nerve, independent of pressure lowering. For example, neuroprotective agents inhibiting the neuron damage induced by excitotoxicity, and drugs that improve the blood flow to the optic nerve, may prove beneficial.

Suggested reading

Alward MD, Wallace LM. *Glaucoma: the requisites in ophthalmology*. New York: Mosby, Inc, 2000.

Choplin NT, Lundy DC (eds). *Atlas of Glaucoma*. London: Martin-Dunitz, 1998.

Eid TM, Spaeth GL. *The glaucomas: concepts and fundamentals*. New York: Lippincott Williams and Wilkins, 2000.

Kanski JJ. *Clinical ophthalmology*, fourth edition. London: Butterworth-Heinemann, 1999.

Ritch R, Shields MB, Krupin T. *The glaucomas*, second edition. New York: Mosby, Inc, 1996.

Shields BM. *Textbook of glaucoma*, fourth edition. Philadelphia: Williams and Wilkins, 1998.

Weingeist TA et al. *Basic and Clinical Science Course, Section 10. Glaucoma: Lifelong education for the Ophthalmologist*. American Academy of Ophthalmology, 1997–98.

2. THE CONCEPT OF 'GLAUCOMA', CLASSIFICATION

Augusto Azuara-Blanco, Richard P Wilson, and Vital P Costa

The concept of 'glaucoma'

The term 'glaucoma' refers to a large number of diseases. The common feature of all glaucomas is a distinctive progressive optic neuropathy, which derives from various risk factors. Glaucomatous optic neuropathy is associated with a gradual loss of the visual field, which can lead to total, irreversible blindness if the disorder is not diagnosed and treated properly.

Classification

The classification of the glaucomas that we propose is based on the underlying abnormality that causes raised intraocular pressure (IOP, Table 2.1). The understanding of the precise mechanism that leads to aqueous obstruction is important for establishing a treatment strategy. The glaucomas are first divided into open-angle glaucomas, angle closure glaucomas, and glaucomas associated with developmental anomalies. These are then subdivided according to specific alterations.

Suggested reading

Shields MB, Ritch R, Krupin T. Classification of the glaucomas. In: Ritch R, Shields MB, Krupin T (eds); The Glaucomas. St Louis, MO: CV Mosby, 1996:717.

Table 2.1 Classification of glaucomas (modified from Shields MB, Ritch R, Krupin T. Classification of the glaucomas. In: Ritch R, Shields MB, Krupin T (eds). The glaucomas. St. Louis, MO: CV Mosby, 1996; p 717)

I. Open-angle glaucomas

- A. Idiopathic
  1. Chronic (primary) open-angle glaucoma
  2. Normal-tension glaucoma
- B. Accumulation of material obstructing the trabecular meshwork
  1. Pigmentary glaucoma
  2. Exfoliative glaucoma
  3. Steroid-induced glaucoma
  4. Inflammatory glaucoma
  5. Lens-induced glaucoma
     a. Phacolytic
     b. Lens-particle
     c. Phacoanaphylactic glaucomas
  6. Ghost cell glaucoma
  7. Neoplastic cell-induced glaucoma
  8. Silicone oil-induced glaucoma
  9. Others
- C. Other abnormalities of the trabecular meshwork
  1. Posner-Schlossman (trabeculitis)
  2. Traumatic glaucoma (angle recession)
  3. Chemical burns
  4. Others
- D. Elevated episcleral venous pressure
  1. Sturge–Weber syndrome
  2. Thyroidopathy
  3. Retrobulbar tumors
  4. Carotid-cavernous fistula
  5. Cavernous sinus thrombosis
  6. Others

II. Angle closure glaucomas

- A. Pupillary block
  1. Primary angle closure glaucoma (acute, sub-acute, chronic, mixed mechanism)
  2. Lens-induced glaucoma
     a. Phacomorphic glaucoma
     b. Lens subluxation
  3. Posterior synechiae
     a. Inflammatory
     b. Pseudophakia
     c. Iris-vitreous

B. Anterior displacement of the iris/lens
    1. Aqueous misdirection
    2. Plateau iris syndrome
    3. Lens-induced glaucoma
        a. Phacomorphic glaucoma
        b. Lens subluxation
    4. Cysts and tumors of the iris and ciliary body
    5. Chorio-retinal abnormalities
        a. Scleral buckle
        b. Suprachoroidal hemorrhage
        c. Tumors
        d. Post panretinal photocoagulation
        e. Retrolenticular contracture (PHPV)
        f. Retinopathy of prematurity
C. Membranes and tissues obstructing outflow
    1. Neovascular glaucoma
    2. Inflammatory glaucoma
    3. ICE syndrome
    4. Epithelial and fibrous downgrowth
    5. Vitreous
    6. Others

III. Developmental anomalies of the anterior chamber angle

A. Isolated anomaly of the anterior chamber angle. Primary congenital glaucoma
B. Glaucoma associated with other ocular or systemic developmental disorders
    1. Aniridia
    2. Axenfeld–Rieger syndrome
    3. Peter's anomaly
    4. Nanophthalmos
    5. Other developmental disorders

3. THE INTRAOCULAR PRESSURE IN GLAUCOMA

Mark R Lesk

In this chapter we discuss methods for measuring intraocular pressure (IOP) and the role of intraocular pressure in the diagnosis and treatment of glaucoma.

Normal intraocular pressure

Based on several large studies, the normal IOP is usually defined as 10–21 mmHg (Figure 3.1). In non-glaucomatous people, the average IOP is roughly 16 mmHg, with a standard deviation of 2.5. However, since many open-angle glaucoma patients have IOPs in this normal range either on screening or at all times when measured, a raised IOP is not necessary for diagnosing open-angle glaucoma (OAG).

Intraocular pressure is subject to a certain degree of variability from day to day and hour to hour. The normal diurnal variation is usually no more than 4 mmHg in normal eyes. Eyes with glaucoma show greater variability, and

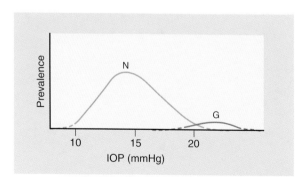

Figure 3.1 Theoretical distribution of intraocular pressure in nonglaucoma (N) and glaucoma populations (G), showing overlap between the two groups. Dotted lines represent uncertainty of extreme values in both populations. Reproduced with permission from Shields MB. Textbook of glaucoma, 4th ed. Baltimore: Williams & Wilkins, 1998: 47.

21

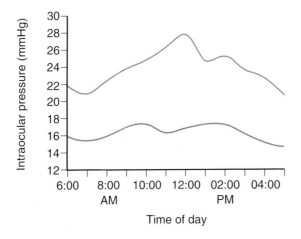

Figure 3.2 Diurnal variation in intraocular pressure.

Normal pressure shows limited variation during the course of a day (bottom curve) while eyes with glaucoma may show considerably more variation (top curve). Reproduced with permission from Choplin NT. Intraocular pressure and its measurement. In: Choplin NT, Lundy DC, eds. Atlas of Glaucoma. London; Martin Dunitz, 1998.

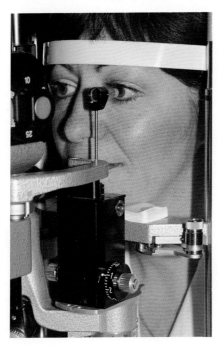

Figure 3.3 Measuring intraocular pressure with the Goldmann tonometer.

The eye is anesthetized and the tear film stained with fluorescein. The instrument is then brought into the appropriate position on the slit lamp and the cobalt blue filter placed in the light path. The slit aperture should be opened widely. The tip of the instrument is gently placed against the cornea, and the image of the tear film is viewed through the biomicroscope. The knob is turned until the inner edges of the semicircles are just touching, indicating that 3.06 mm of corneal flattening has been attained, corresponding to the intraocular pressure. The reading on the knob is multiplied by ten to obtain the pressure reading.

patients may have spikes of IOP (that occur most commonly in the morning) while measuring within the normal range other times (Figure 3.2).

Methods of measuring intraocular pressure

The most widely used and generally accepted gold standard for measuring the IOP is Goldmann tonometry (Figure 3.3). Goldmann detemined that when an applanation surface diameter was 3.06 mm in a human eye with 520 µm corneal thickness, then the surface tension and the resistance of the cornea were balanced and could be ignored. Thus, during tonometry, the objective is to applanate a diameter of 3.06 mm. This is achieved when the inner border of the fluorescein rings are in contact at the mid-point of their pulsations (Figure 3.4).

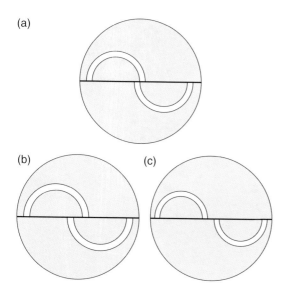

Figure 3.4 Tear film meniscus. Appearance of tear film meniscus as viewed through the Goldmann tonometer during applanation tonometry.

(a) Correct appearance of the mires when the applied force to the cornea is equal to the intraocular pressure. (b) Appearance of the mires when the applied force is greater than the intraocular pressure or the instrument is pushed too far into the eye, indicating that the cornea has been overflattened. (c) Appearance of the mires when the applied force is less then the intraocular pressure, indicating that the cornea has been underflattened. Reproduced with permission from Choplin NT. Intraocular pressure and its measurement. In: Choplin NT, Lundy DC, eds. Atlas of Glaucoma. London; Martin Dunitz, 1998.

Table 3.1 Common sources of error in the application of Goldman tonometry (and direction of error)

Contact of tonometer with lids or lashes (↑)
Pressure by operator's finger on globe (through eyelid) (↑)
Fluorescein ring too thick (↑) or thin (↓)
Absence of fluorescein (↓)
Prolonged tonometer contact (↓)

Table 3.2 Common sources of error in Goldmann tonometry related to biological variability (and direction of error)

Raised (↑) or decreased (↓) central corneal thickness
Corneal epithelial or stromal edema (↓)
Corneal scarring (↑)
Increased venous pressure from tight clothing (↑)
Valsalva maneuver (↑ or ↓)
Ciliary muscle contraction (↑ if acute, ↓ if sustained)
Restrictive ocular myopathy or orbital disease (↑)
Blepharospasm (↑)

At this time, the value in grams on the tension knob, when multiplied by ten, is equivalent to the IOP in mmHg.

Interobserver variability of Goldmann tonometry has been estimated at 0–3 mmHg. The two general sources of error with Goldmann tonometry can be categorized as those caused by faults in the application of the technique (Table 3.1) and those related to biological variability of the human eye and orbit, both normal and pathological (Table 3.2).

Of particular note is the error induced by normal or post-surgical variability of the central corneal thickness (CCT). CCT is measured with an optical or ultrasound pachymeter. Although the Goldmann tonometer is calibrated for a CCT of 520 μm, in one large study of normal subjects the CCT ranged from 427–620 μm with a mean of 537 μm. It is estimated that for eyes with glaucoma or ocular hypertension, Goldmann tonometry *overestimates* the IOP by 2–3 mmHg for every 50 μm thickness above average. Thus many ocular hypertensive patients, whose IOP may have been overestimated because of raised CCT, may be reclassified as normal once the CCT is measured. Alternately, patients with thin corneas may have their IOPs *underestimated*, although the correction factor is unlikely to exceed 4–5 mmHg. After refractive surgery, the CCT is altered and tonometry results must be interpreted with caution. Underestimation of the IOP by 2–4 mmHg is probably common after LASIK.

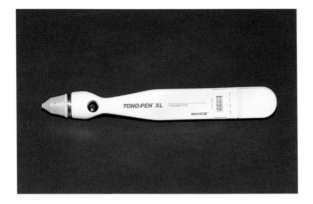

Figure 3.5 The Tonopen tonometer.

This miniaturized electronic applanation tonometer is battery powered and can be used in any position. It is very useful for measuring intraocular pressure in patients who cannot sit at a slit lamp. It is also useful for measuring pressures in patients with irregular corneas, since the applanation area is much smaller than that of the Goldmann instrument.

The Perkins tonometer is a portable device similar to the Goldmann tonometer. Like the other portable devices, it is useful in situations where a patient cannot be seated at a slit lamp, such as bedside examinations, the operating room, nursing homes, remote areas, and mass screenings.

The Tonopen (Figure 3.5) is an automated hand-held applanation tonometer based on the MacKay-Marg tonometer. It is particularly useful when the cornea is scarred or irregular, when Goldmann tonometry may yield distorted and variable fluorescein rings that are difficult to interpret.

Non-contact tonometers applanate the cornea with a puff of air. Measurement errors are greater in patients who squeeze their eyelids or who blink rapidly in response to the startling jet of air, and in eyes with moderately raised IOPs. Although there is no direct contact between the instrument and the eye, a tear film aerosol is produced that may contain infectious material. The advantage of this instrument is that, since there is no direct contact with the eye, it can be operated by non-medical personnel.

The Schiøtz tonometer (Figure 3.6) works by the principle of indentation, whereby a small weight is placed on the cornea and the IOP is estimated by the degree of indentation. Higher Schiøtz scale readings indicate lower IOPs. The conversion is made using a chart kept with the tonometer. The Schiøtz tonometer is an accurate and portable mechanical instrument that is simple to use. It will give errors in eyes with abnormal ocular rigidity, such as eyes with longstanding glaucoma or high hyperopia (overestimations of IOP), or with

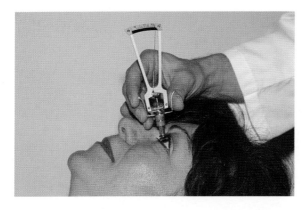

Figure 3.6 Measurement of intraocular pressure with a Schiotz tonometer.
The patient is placed in the supine position and topical anesthetic applied. The patient is instructed to look straight ahead or fixate on a point on the ceiling with the fellow eye. Holding the instrument by the handles, it is gently applied perpendicularly to the cornea until the footplate rests on the cornea. The plunger, with the attached load weight, pushes down on the cornea and indents it to the amount allowed by the resistance of the intraocular pressure. This causes the jewel-mounted plunger to push back on the convex hammer, causing the pointer to deflect off zero on the inclined scale. Since the lever ratio is 1:20, the reading corresponds to the amount of corneal indentation $\times$ 0.05 mm. Once the scale reading has been determined, the intraocular pressure is read from the calibration chart.

myopia, strong miotic therapy or retinal detachment surgery (underestimations of IOP).

Role of intraocular pressure in the diagnosis of glaucoma

Intraocular pressure has three roles in the diagnosis of glaucoma.

1 In ocular hypertension, raised IOP is the primary criterion for making the diagnosis in an eye that has normal optic nerve heads and normal visual fields.
2 In primary open angle glaucoma (POAG), raised IOP is not required to make the diagnosis; typical glaucomatous ONH changes and visual field changes are required. Diurnal IOP curves are sometimes useful to deter-

mine whether the patient shows significant, potentially dangerous, pressure spikes during the course of the day and to establish a more meaningful 'Tmax'—the patient's maximal recorded iOP. Such testing can also help classify patients as normal tension glaucoma patients (as opposed to POAG), although this distinction is of relatively little practical significance.

3   In congenital and secondary glaucoma, the diagnosis is usually based on the presence of raised IOP. The presence of glaucomatous optic nerve atrophy simply confirms the diagnosis and makes cases more severe.

Role of intraocular pressure in the treatment of glaucoma

Intraocular pressure has a central role in the treatment of all forms of glaucoma. It is the main risk factor for glaucoma and can be lowered with medical or surgical treatment (see Chapter 15). Almost every treatment offered to glaucoma patients is aimed at reducing the IOP.

Ideally, a newly diagnosed patient' intraocular pressure should be measured several times during a day to determine that patient's maximal untreated IOP, also known as 'Tmax'. Using the Tmax, the state of the optic nerve and visual field, and the patient's risk factors for deteriorating, a therapeutic objective or 'target pressure' (Tgoal) can be established. All subsequent therapy is aimed at achieving that Tgoal. Once Tgoal is achieved, patients are followed for signs of deterioration of the optic nerve or visual field. If there is evidence of deterioration then a new, lower, Tgoal is set, usually by a further 20–30% intraocular pressure reduction.

Calculation of initial Tgoal, the target therapeutic intraocular pressure

Several formulas have been described to calculate the 'target pressure' (Tgoal). Here, we propose one of them. In a three-step process, the Tgoal may be calculated independently for each eye. To calculate Tgoal, the maximum known intraocular pressure (Tmax) is first reduced by 'its own percent' (see footnote). In other words, if Tmax is 20 mmHg, it is reduced by 20%, if Tmax is 35 mmHg it is reduced by 35%, etc. The second step is to further reduce the Tgoal by a percent equivalent to the mean defect or mean deficit on automated perimetry. If automated perimetry cannot be done then the clinician can estimate what might be expected if it were to be performed (i.e. an M.D. of 10 db in moderately advanced glaucoma, or an M.D. of 20 db in advanced glaucoma). The final step is to further reduce the Tgoal based on the patient's risk factors for losing significant vision during his or her lifetime. These risk factors include family history of blindness from glaucoma, loss of fixation in the contralateral eye, black race, young age, presence of migraines, and presence of other vascular disease. An additional 10–15% reduction in the Tgoal may be required if one or more risk factors are present. An example is given in the box.

Calculation of Tgoal, the target IOP

A 52-year-old man of African descent presents with newly diagnosed OAG. He has treated systemic hypertension. His Tmax is 27 mmHg O.D. and 29 mmHg O.S. based on three measurements before starting treament. His visual acuity is 6/6 O.D., but he has lost fixation O.S. Cup/disc ratio is 0.8 O.D. and 0.9 + O.S. The mean defect on Humphrey automated perimetry is –8 db O.D.

To calculate Tgoal for the right eye, begin by reducing 27 mmHg by 27%:

$$27 - (27 \times 0.27) = 27 - 7.29 \approx 19.7$$

Secondly, adjust for the 8 db mean defect by an additional 8% reduction:

$$19.7 - (27 \times 0.08) = 19.7 - 2.16 \approx 17.5$$

Thirdly, adjust for risk factors. In this case race, age, status of the contralateral eye and vascular disease are relevant. An adjustment by approximately 10% or 2.7mmHg is appropriate.

$$17.5 - 2.7 = 14.8$$

Our goal IOP, Tgoal, is around 15 mmHg for the right eye.

The formula, adapted from that used for calculating Tgoal in the Advanced Glaucoma Intervention Study (AGIS) is:

$$\text{Tgoal} = \text{Tmax} - (\text{Tmax} \times (\text{Tmax}/100))$$

Suggested reading

Advanced Glaucoma Intervention Study. 2. Visual field test scoring and reliability. *Ophthalmology* 1994;**101**(8):1445–55.

Boothe WA Lee DA, Parek WC, Pettit TH. The Tono-Pen: a manometric study. *Invest Ophthalmol Vis Sci* 1987;**28**(suppl):134.

Damji KF, Munger R. Influence of central corneal thickness on applanation intgaocular pressure. *J Glaucoma* 2000;**9**(3):205–7.

Goldmann H. Un nouveau tomètre d'applanation. *Bull Soc Ophthalmol Fr* 1955;**67**:474–8.

Lewis RA. Refractive surgery and the glaucoma patient. *Ophthalmology* 2000;**107**(9):1621–2.

Leydhecker W, Akiyama K, Neumann HG. Der intraokulare Druck gesunderMenschAugen. *Klin Mbl Augenheilk* 1958;**133**:662.

Phelps CD, Phelps GK. Measurement of intraocular pressure: a study of its reproducibility. *Graefes Arch Clin Exp Ophthalmol* 1976;**198**:39.

Shah S. Accurate intraocular pressure measurement – the myth of modern ophthalmology? *Ophthalmology*, 2000;**107**(10):1805–7.

Shields MB. The non-contact tonometer: its value and limitations. *Survey Opthalmol* 1980;**24**:211.

Sommer A, Tielsch JM, Katz J et al. Relationship between intraocular pressure and primary open angle glaucoma among white and black Americans. The Baltimore Eye Survey. *Arch Ophthalmol* 1991;**109**:1090–5.

Stamper RL, Lieberman MF, Drake MV. Intraocular Pressure. In: Becker–Shaffer's Diagnosis and Therapy of the Glaucomas, 7th edn. Stamper RL, Lieberman MF, Drake MV (eds). 1999, Mosby, St Louis, 65–82.

Whitacre MM, Stein R. Sources of Error with use of Goldmann-type tonometers. *Surv Ophthalmol* 1993;**38**(1):1–30.

Wolfs RCW, Klaver CCW, Vingerling JR et al. Distribution of central corneal thickness and its association with intraocular pressure: The Rotterdam Study. *Am J Ophthalmol* 1997;**123**:767–72.

Table 3.1 Common sources of error in the application of Goldman tonometry (and direction of error)

Contact of tonometer with lids or lashes (↑)
Pressure by operator's finger on globe (through eyelid) (↑)
Fluorescein ring too thick (↑) or thin (↓)
Absence of fluorescein (↓)
Prolonged tonometer contact (↓)

Table 3.2 Common sources of error in Goldmann tonometry related to biological variability (and direction of error)

Raised (↑) or decreased (↓) central corneal thickness
Corneal epithelial or stromal edema (↓)
Corneal scarring (↑)
Increased venous pressure from tight clothing (↑)
Valsalva maneuver (↑ or ↓)
Ciliary muscle contraction (↑ if acute, ↓ if sustained)
Restrictive ocular myopathy or orbital disease (↑)
Blepharospasm (↑)

At this time, the value in grams on the tension knob, when multiplied by ten, is equivalent to the IOP in mmHg.

Interobserver variability of Goldmann tonometry has been estimated at 0–3 mmHg. The two general sources of error with Goldmann tonometry can be categorized as those caused by faults in the application of the technique (Table 3.1) and those related to biological variability of the human eye and orbit, both normal and pathological (Table 3.2).

Of particular note is the error induced by normal or post-surgical variability of the central corneal thickness (CCT). CCT is measured with an optical or ultrasound pachymeter. Although the Goldmann tonometer is calibrated for a CCT of 520 μm, in one large study of normal subjects the CCT ranged from 427–620 μm with a mean of 537 μm. It is estimated that for eyes with glaucoma or ocular hypertension, Goldmann tonometry *overestimates* the IOP by 2–3 mmHg for every 50 μm thickness above average. Thus many ocular hypertensive patients, whose IOP may have been overestimated because of raised CCT, may be reclassified as normal once the CCT is measured. Alternately, patients with thin corneas may have their IOPs *underestimated*, although the correction factor is unlikely to exceed 4–5 mmHg. After refractive surgery, the CCT is altered and tonometry results must be interpreted with caution. Underestimation of the IOP by 2–4 mmHg is probably common after LASIK.

patients may have spikes of IOP (that occur most commonly in the morning) while measuring within the normal range other times (Figure 3.2).

Methods of measuring intraocular pressure

The most widely used and generally accepted gold standard for measuring the IOP is Goldmann tonometry (Figure 3.3). Goldmann detemined that when an applanation surface diameter was 3.06 mm in a human eye with 520 μm corneal thickness, then the surface tension and the resistance of the cornea were balanced and could be ignored. Thus, during tonometry, the objective is to applanate a diameter of 3.06 mm. This is achieved when the inner border of the fluorescein rings are in contact at the mid-point of their pulsations (Figure 3.4).

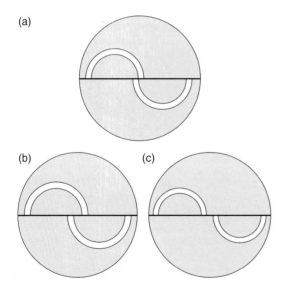

Figure 3.4 Tear film meniscus. Appearance of tear film meniscus as viewed through the Goldmann tonometer during applanation tonometry.

(a) Correct appearance of the mires when the applied force to the cornea is equal to the intraocular pressure. (b) Appearance of the mires when the applied force is greater than the intraocular pressure or the instrument is pushed too far into the eye, indicating that the cornea has been overflattened. (c) Appearance of the mires when the applied force is less then the intraocular pressure, indicating that the cornea has been underflattened. Reproduced with permission from Choplin NT. Intraocular pressure and its measurement. In: Choplin NT, Lundy DC, eds. Atlas of Glaucoma. London; Martin Dunitz, 1998.

4. ANTERIOR CHAMBER ANGLE EXAMINATION: GONIOSCOPY AND ULTRASOUND BIOMICROSCOPY

Celso Tello, Jeffrey M Liebmann and Robert Ritch

Knowledge of the anatomy and pathology of the anterior segment is critical for the accurate diagnosis and effective treatment of glaucoma. Examination of anterior segment structures and their relation can be done with complementary techniques including slit-lamp biomicroscopy, gonioscopy and ultrasound biomicroscopy (UBM).

Slit-lamp biomicroscopy provides a direct view of the cornea, lens, iris, conjunctiva and sclera. However, slit-lamp biomicroscopy does not allow direct visualization of the anterior chamber angle, which is best achieved with gonioscopy. Indentation gonioscopy permits dynamic evaluation of the angle and the assessment of appositional or synechial closure. These clinical techniques may be complemented by new, reliable, high resolution imaging systems, which can enhance our understanding of ocular anatomy and pathophysiology.

High frequency, high resolution UBM (Paradigm Medical Industries, Inc., Salt Lake City, Utah, USA) produces high resolution in vivo images of the anterior segment. This technology uses high frequency transducers to assess anatomical relations of structures within the anterior segment. The purpose of this review is to discuss the role of gonioscopy and UBM in the diagnosis and management of the glaucomas.

Anatomy of the anterior chamber angle

The anterior chamber angle can be described as a recess bordered posteriorly by the anterior surface of the peripheral iris and anteriorly by the peripheral corneal endothelium, Schwalbe's line, trabecular meshwork, scleral spur, and ciliary body band (Figure 4.1).

The iris root inserts into the anterior face of the ciliary body. The iris offers little resistance to a relative increase or decrease in pressure within the anterior or posterior chambers, allowing the iris to take on a concave or convex appearance when there is an alteration in the pressure gradient between the two chambers. The trabecular meshwork is the main outflow pathway of aqueous humor. It originates in the deep layers of the cornea anteriorly and extends to the scleral spur posteriorly.

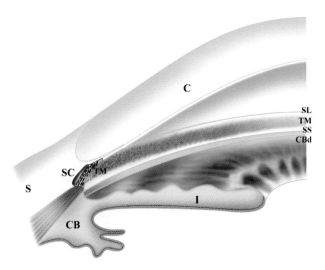

Figure 4.1 Anterior chamber angle anatomy. SL = Schwalbe's line; TM = trabecular meshwork; SS = scleral spur; CBd = ciliary board; SC = Schlemm's canal; I = iris; S = sclera; CB = ciliary body. Reproduced with permission from Achache F, Anatomical features of outflow pathway. In *Non-penetrating Glaucoma Surgery*, Mermoud A and Shaaraway T. Martin Dunitz, London, 2001.

Schwalbe's line is a ring formed by circumferentially directed bundles of connective tissue supported by collagen and elastic material, and marks the peripheral extent of Descemet's membrane. The longitudinal muscle of the ciliary body inserts into the scleral spur and is located at the posterior border of the trabecular meshwork.

Gonioscopy: equipment and technique

Gonioscopy allows visualization of the anterior chamber angle by using direct or indirect contact lenses. The principle of this technique is based on changing the refraction of light (coming from the anterior chamber angle towards the cornea), by replacing the air surface component of the air–tear film interface by a medium of higher refractive index, such as a goniolens (Figure 4.2).

Direct gonioscopy is performed with a Koeppe lens (50-diopter concave lens), a binocular microscope and a fiberoptic illuminator. This contact lens is placed on the anesthetized eye with the patient in the supine position (Figure 4.3A). The space between the lens and the cornea is filled with an optical coupling agent such as saline solution or methylcellulose. The Koeppe lens provides a direct and panoramic view of the angle, and can be used to visualize the anterior chamber angle during procedures such as goniotomy.

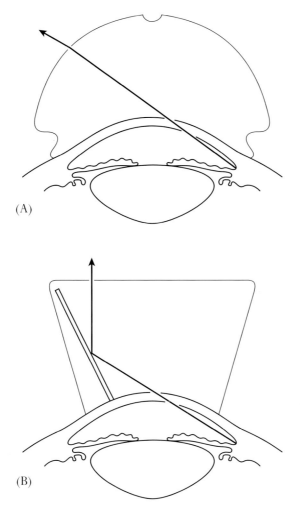

Figure 4.2 (A) Direct gonioscopy performed with Koeppe lens. Fig. 4.2a Reproduced with permission from Ritch R, Shields MB, Krupin. The Glaucomas. Second edition, Mosby, St Louis, 1996 (page 460). (B) Indirect gonioscopy performed with a goniolens with one or more mirrors. From: Kolker AE, Hetherington J, eds. Becker-Shaffer's Diagnosis and Therapy of the Glaucomas. 5th ed. St Louis: CV Mosby Co; 1983.

Indirect gonioscopy is performed with goniolenses containing one or more mirrors (Goldmann, Zeiss, Posner, Sussman). This technique can be accomplished with the patient in the seated position at the slit-lamp (Figure 4.3B). Indirect gonioscopy provides an inverted image of the opposite angle. To improve

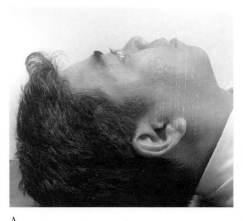

A

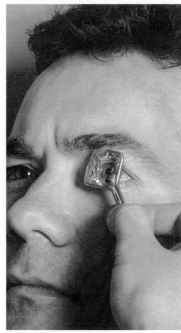

Figure 4.3 (A) Koeppe lens with patient in supine position. (B) Zeiss lens with patient in sitting position.

B

visibility of the angle, the mirror can be tilted toward the angle under examination, or the patient can be asked to look toward the mirror.

The Goldmann lens requires an optical coupling between the cornea and the lens. A disadvantage of this lens is that posterior pressure may indent the sclera and falsely narrow the angle. On the other hand, the four-mirror Zeiss lens and other lenses (Posner, Sussman) have a smaller area of contact than the Goldmann lens and have almost the same radius of curvature as the cornea, which allows the tear film to function as the optical coupling agent. When using these small diameter lenses, pressure over the cornea will displace aqueous from the center of the anterior chamber into the periphery, dislocating the iris posteriorly and falsely opening the anterior chamber angle. Indentation gonioscopy relies on this phenomenon and is crucial for the differential diagnosis of the angle-closure glaucomas (Figure 4.4).

During gonioscopy, the examiner should be able to identify the structures of the anterior chamber angle (Figure 4.1). Using a narrow slit beam at an oblique angle, two linear reflections can be identified: one from the external surface of the cornea and its junction with the sclera, the other from the internal surface of the cornea. The two reflections meet at Schwalbe's line. The slit of light appears above Schwalbe's line as a three-dimensional parallelepiped of light.

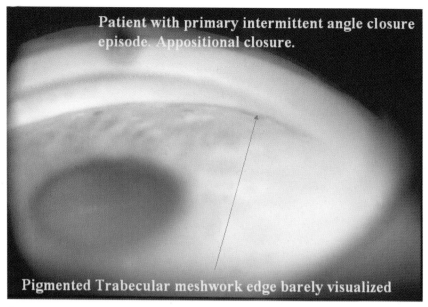

A

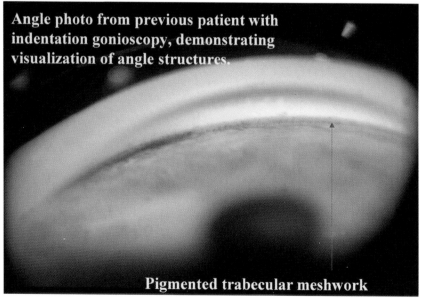

B

Figure 4.4 (A) Gonioscopy without indentation, angle closure, no angle structures are seen. (B) Gonioscopy with indentation, angle structures are seen (same patient from Figure 3.4A). Courtesy of José Morales MD, Associate Professor, Texas Tech University.

Posterior to Schwalbe's line is the trabecular meshwork. The pigmented posterior band corresponds to the filtering portion of the meshwork. The scleral spur appears as a thin, white band located between the trabecular meshwork and the ciliary face. Normal blood vessels are distributed either radially along the iris or circumferentially within the ciliary body face. Vessels that cross the scleral spur onto the trabecular meshwork are abnormal. The *parallelepiped method* described by Palmberg is extremely useful for identifying landmarks in eyes with closed angles or open angles with no trabecular meshwork pigmentation.

Once the gonioscopic landmarks have been identified, angle pathology can be recognized. This includes *thickening and anterior displacement of Schwalbe's line* (posterior embryotoxon), *pathological trabecular meshwork pigmentation* (pigment dispersion syndrome, exfoliation syndrome, tumors), *peripheral anterior synechiae* (adhesions of iris to the trabecular meshwork) [which should be differentiated from *iris processes* (lacy cords of uveal tissue that may extend to the trabecular meshwork), *neovascular membranes* (trunk vessels rise across the scleral spur which branch out on the surface of the trabecular meshwork)], *blood in Schlemm's canal* (when episcleral venous pressure exceeds IOP), *exfoliative material, Sampaolesi's line, uveal tumors* (flat or elevated lesions), *angle dysgenesis, angle recession* (traumatic separation of the longitudinal and circular fibers of the ciliary muscle), *cyclodialysis cleft* (separation of the ciliary muscle from the scleral spur), *foreign bodies* and, most importantly, determination of the degree of *angle aperture.*

When assessing a patient for anterior chamber angle occludability, it is important to perform indentation gonioscopy in a completely darkened room, using the smallest square of light for a slit beam to avoid stimulating the pupillary light reflex. With the lights on and a narrow, short slit beam off axis, the quadrant of the angle to be assessed is first examined with the Zeiss four-mirror lens, with no pressure on the cornea and with the patient looking sufficiently far in the direction of the mirror that the examiner can see as deeply into the angle as possible. The narrowest quadrant, usually the superior angle (inferior mirror) is the one to observe.

The gonioscopic grading systems in use today have been described by Shaffer and Spaeth. The most common system used is the one proposed by Shaffer, who described the angle between the trabecular meshwork and the iris as follows:

Grade IV.   Iridocorneal angle of 40 degrees or more.
Grade III. Iridocorneal angle greater than 20 but less than 40 degrees.
Grade II.   Iridocorneal angle of 20 degrees.
Grade I.   Iridocorneal angle of 10 degrees.
Slit.   Iridocorneal angle of less than 10 degrees.
O.   The iris is against the trabecular meshwork.

Spaeth's classification expands Shaffer's to include a description of the angular approach, the peripheral iris contour, and the site of iris insertion. *Angularity of the anterior chamber* is graded as the angle determined by the corneal endothelium surface and the anterior surface of the iris, measured at the Schwalbe's line. (Figure 4.5A). *Peripheral iris configuration* is called 's' when there is a plateau-configuration with an anterior convexity and sudden drop to a flat iris centrally; 'q' when there is posterior concavity; and 'r' when the iris is flat or 'regular'

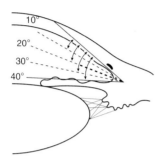

A

Figure 4.5 Spaeth gonioscopic grading system, based on three variables: (A) angle width of the anterior chamber angle; (B) configuration of the peripheral iris, and (C), site of iris insertion. Fig. 4.5 Reproduced with permission from Shields MB. Textbook of Glaucoma. Fourth edition, Williams & Wilkins, Baltimore, 1998 (page 184).

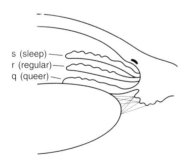

B

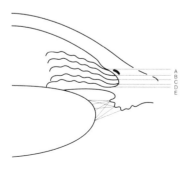

C

37

(Figure 4.5B). *Iris insertion sites* are graded as follows: A, anterior to Schwalbe's line; B, just anterior to the posterior trabecular meshwork; C, just anterior to the ciliary body (scleral spur is visible); D, ciliary body visible; and E, 1 mm or more of ciliary body visible (Figure 4.5C).

Ultrasound biomicroscopy: equipment and technique

High frequency ultrasound biomicroscopy (UBM) is a non-invasive diagnostic technique that uses high frequency transducers to provide high resolution, in vivo imaging of the anterior segment. The structures surrounding the posterior chamber, including the ciliary body, iridolenticular relationship and zonules, previously hidden from clinical observation, can be imaged and their normal anatomical relations assessed. Pathological changes involving anterior segment architecture can be qualitatively and quantitatively assessed.

The currently available commercial unit operates at 50 MHz and provides lateral and axial resolution of approximately 50 μm and 25 μm, respectively. Tissue penetration is approximately 4–5 mm. The scanner produces a 5 × 5-mm field with 256 vertical image lines (or A-scans) at a scan rate of 8 frames per second. The technique of UBM has been reported in detail elsewhere. Ultrasonography measurements are strongly dependent on the examiner's technique and experience. The distance from the center of the anterior chamber, plane of section, and the orientation of the probe may affect the apparent structural configuration of the anterior segment.

Quantitative assessment of anterior segment relations using the information contained in UBM scans requires a more sophisticated approach. Pavlin and colleagues described and quantified normal values for anterior segment anatomy, although this approach is limited by interobserver variability. Factors that contribute to the variability of UBM image acquisition include room illumination, fixation, and accommodative effort, each of them affecting anterior segment anatomy by altering the pupillary size. These variables should be held constant, particularly when quantitative information is being gathered. In our laboratory, patients are asked to fixate with the fellow eye at a ceiling-mounted target to minimize changes in accommodation and eye position. Room illumination is held constant. Since the probe is in constant motion during scanning, a soft contact lens may be used to prevent potential corneal injury.

Ultrasound biomicroscopy and the normal eye

Familiarity with the ultrasound biomicroscopic appearance of normal ocular anatomy is important for recognizing pathological changes. In the normal eye,

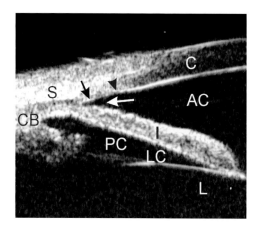

Figure 4.6 Ultrasound biomicroscopy of a normal eye. The cornea (C), anterior chamber (AC), angle recess (white arrow), iris (I), lens (L), lens capsule (LC), posterior chamber (PC), scleral spur (black arrow), Schwalbe's line (arrowhead) sclera (S), and ciliary body (CB) are visible.

the cornea, anterior chamber, posterior chamber, iris, ciliary body, and anterior lens surface can be easily recognized.

Since the trabecular meshwork itself cannot be visualized with UBM, identification of the scleral spur during imaging localizes its posterior extent. In a UBM image, the scleral spur can be seen as the innermost point of the line separating the ciliary body and the sclera at its point of contact with the anterior chamber. The trabecular meshwork is located directly anterior to this structure and posterior to Schwalbe's line (Figure 4.6).

Ultrasound biomicroscopy and ocular pathology

Angle-closure glaucoma

Accurate diagnosis of the angle-closure glaucomas is critical to both their detection and treatment. Although gonioscopic assessment of the anterior chamber angle with a Goldmann or Koeppe lens provides information about angle anatomy, clinical examination of the angle with the Zeiss indentation gonioprism permits dynamic evaluation of the angle configuration and allows the clinician to differentiate synechial from appositional closure.

Angle-closure glaucomas are best classified according to the anatomical findings produced by the sequence of events that results in iridotrabecular contact. Forces acting at four anatomical levels may alter the configuration of the angle and may predispose to angle closure glaucoma. These include the iris (pupillary block), the ciliary body (plateau iris), the lens (phacomorphic glaucoma), and forces posterior to the lens (malignant glaucoma).

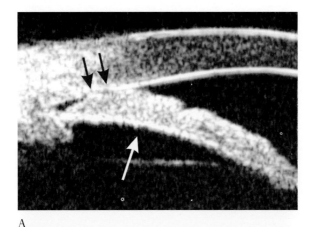

A

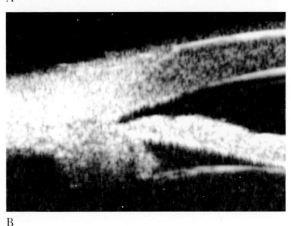

B

Figure 4.7 (A) The iris has a convex configuration (white arrow) in pupillary block angle closure because of the relative pressure differential between the posterior chamber and the anterior chamber. The angle is closed (black arrows). (B) After laser iridotomy, aqueous has free access to the anterior chamber and the pressure gradient is eliminated. The iris assumes a flat (planar) configuration and the angle opens.

Pupillary block

Relative pupillary block is an impedance to the flow of aqueous humor from the posterior chamber to the anterior chamber. The accumulation of aqueous in the posterior chamber forces the peripheral iris anteriorly, causing anterior iris bowing, narrowing of the angle, and acute or chronic angle-closure glaucoma (Figure 4.7). Ultrasound biomicroscopy should be done in darkened conditions to assess the anterior chamber angle configuration during pupillary dilation. In fact, our current provocative test of choice uses UBM under light and dark room conditions.

Plateau iris

Plateau iris configuration results from a large or anteriorly positioned pars plicata that mechanically holds the ciliary body against the trabecular meshwork

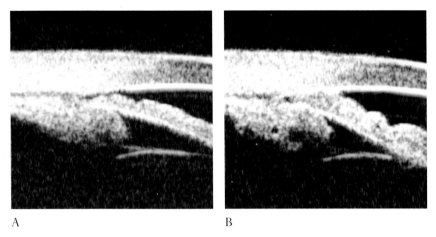

A   B

Figure 4.8 (A) In plateau iris syndrome, the angle is narrow secondary to a large or anteriorly positioned ciliary body. (B) In darkened conditions the angle closes.

(Figure 4.8). Plateau iris *syndrome* refers to the development of angle closure, either spontaneously or after pupillary dilation, in an eye with plateau iris configuration despite the presence of a patent iridectomy or iridotomy. Acute angle-closure glaucoma may develop. The extent or the 'height' to which the plateau rises determines whether or not the angle will close completely with a rise in IOP (complete plateau iris syndrome) or only partially without a rise in IOP (incomplete plateau iris syndrome).

In pseudoplateau iris, the clinical appearance of the anterior chamber angle is similar to that which is seen in plateau iris syndrome, although the anterior displacement of the peripheral iris is not caused by an enlarged or anteriorly positioned ciliary body. Cysts of the iris and/or ciliary body neuroepithelium most often cause this disorder (Figure 4.9).

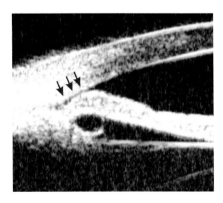

Figure 4.9 Pseudoplateau iris caused by iridociliary cysts. (black arrows).

Lens-related angle-closure

Progressive lens intumescence leads to an increase in its axial length, iridolenticular contact and resistance to aqueous flow from the posterior to the anterior chamber. Accumulation of aqueous in the posterior chamber will cause bowing of the peripheral iris and narrowing of the anterior chamber angle. In cases where the swelling of the lens is severe, the iris may be mechanically pushed against the trabecular meshwork.

Malignant glaucoma

Malignant glaucoma, also known as ciliary block or aqueous misdirection, is characterized by raised IOP, shallow anterior chamber, patent iridectomy, and unremarkable posterior segment anatomy by ophthalmoscopy and B-scan ultrasonography.

The anatomy and pathophysiology of malignant glaucoma remain unclear. Shaffer proposed that aqueous flow is diverted into the vitreous cavity. He attributed the aqueous misdirection to an abnormal vitreociliary relationship and later coined the term 'ciliary block glaucoma'. Epstein and colleagues theorized that in malignant glaucoma there is thickening of the anterior hyaloid, with posterior diversion of aqueous. The accumulation of aqueous within the posterior segment forces the ciliary body and hyaloid face anteriorly, shallowing the anterior chamber and causing a secondary angle closure glaucoma.

We have identified at least two distinct mechanisms that may cause what is usually called postoperative malignant glaucoma. In the first group, the ciliary body is detached and rotated anteriorly, causing angle closure (Figure 4.10A). In the second group there is aqueous misdirection without UBM evidence of ciliary body detachment (Figure 4.10B).

Open-angle glaucomas

Pigment dispersion syndrome

Pigment dispersion syndrome is an autosomal dominant disorder in which mechanical friction between the posterior iris surface and anterior zonular bundles results in disruption of iris pigment epithelial cells. Liberated pigment particles accumulate throughout the anterior segment, resulting in trabecular dysfunction and raised IOP. The iris tends to have a concave configuration on gonioscopy, and its insertion on the ciliary face is typically posterior. UBM illustrates a widely open angle associated with a peripheral iris concavity (Figure 4.11).

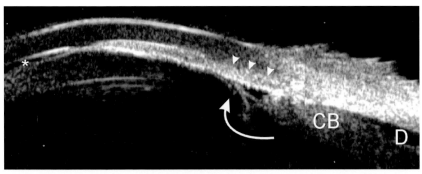

A

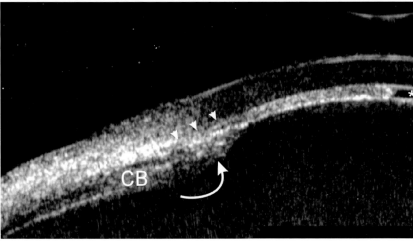

B

Figure 4.10 (A) Malignant glaucoma caused by ciliary body (CB) detachment (D) and anterior rotation. The anterior chamber (asterisk) is flat and the lens–iris diaphragm (curved arrow) is rotated forward to cause mechanical angle-closure. (white arrowheads). (B) Aqueous misdirection with absence of ciliary body (CB) detachment. The anterior chamber (asterisk) is flat and the lens–iris diaphragm (curved arrow) is rotated forward to cause mechanical angle-closure. (white arrowheads).

Juvenile primary open-angle glaucoma

Juvenile primary open-angle glaucoma, defined as primary open-angle glaucoma appearing between the ages of 10 and 35 years, is usually familial and accompanied by markedly raised IOP. UBM investigation of these patients showed the trabecular meshwork to be shorter than in eyes with similar degrees of myopia.

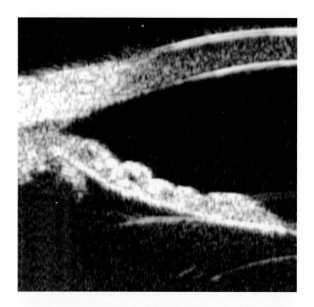

Figure 4.11 In pigment dispersion syndrome the iris configuration is typically concave.

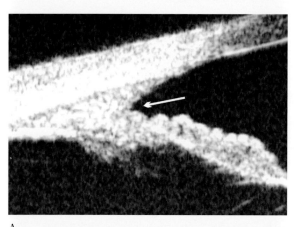

A

Figure 4.12 (A) In angle recession, the injury causes a tear between the longitudinal and circular fibers of the ciliary muscle (white arrow). (B) In a cyclodialysis cleft, there is a detachment of the ciliary muscle from the scleral spur (white arrow).

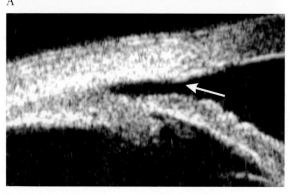

B

Ocular trauma

Ocular trauma may result in diverse anterior segment pathologies including hyphema, cyclodialysis, and angle recession, among others that may cause glaucoma. Gonioscopic assessment may be limited in patients with hyphema or hypotony secondary to a cyclodialysis cleft. UBM plays an important role in the clarification of the status of the anterior chamber angle under these conditions (Figure 4.12).

Ultrasound biomicroscopy and other ocular disorders

Ultrasound biomicroscopy is useful for the diagnosis of pathologies involving the ciliary body and pars plana such as tumors, as well as for the assessment of the anterior segment in eyes with opaque media such as Peters' anomaly, sclerocornea, and corneal opacification.

Summary

Assessment of the anterior chamber angle by use of complementary techniques including slit-lamp biomicroscopy, gonioscopy and ultrasound biomicroscopy is an important step for an accurate diagnosis and effective treatment of different types of glaucomas and other pathologies involving the anterior chamber angle.

Acknowledgements

Supported by a grant from the New York Glaucoma Research Institute, New York, NY, USA.

Suggested reading

Azuara-Blanco A, Spaeth GL, Araujo SV et al. Plateau iris syndrome associated with multiple ciliary body cysts. Report of three cases. *Arch Ophthalmol* 1996;**114**:666–8.

Epstein DL, Hashimoto JM, Anderson PJ et al. Experimental perfusions through the anterior and vitreous chambers with possible relationships to malignant glaucoma. *Am J Ophthalmol* 1979;**88**:1078.

Forbes M. Gonioscopy with corneal indentation: a method for distinguishing between appositional closure and synechial closure. *Arch Ophthalmol* 1966;**76**:488–97.

Karickhoff JR. Pigmentary dispersion syndrome and pigmentary glaucoma: a new mechanism concept, a new treatment, and a new technique. *Ophthalmic Surg* 1992;**23**:269–77.

Kolker AE, Hetherington J Jr. Becker-Shaffer's diagnosis and therapy of the glaucomas. St Louis; Mosby, 1976.

Liebmann JM, Tello C, Chew S-J et al. Prevention of blinking alters iris configuration in pigment dispersion syndrome and in normal eyes. *Ophthalmology* 1995;**102**:446–55.

Lowe RF. Plateau iris. *Aust J Ophthalmol* 1981;**9**:71–3.

Ludwig K, Wegscheider E, Hoops JP et al. In vivo imaging of the human zonular apparatus with high-resolution ultrasound biomicroscopy. *Graefes Arch Clin Exp Ophthalmol* 1999;**237**:361–71.

Marigo FA, Finger PT, McCormick SA et al. Anterior segment implantation cysts. Ultrasound biomicroscopy with histopathologic correlation. *Arch Ophthalmol* 1998;**116**:1569–75.

Martinez-Bello C, Capeans C, Sanchez-Salorio M. Ultrasound biomicroscopy in the diagnosis of supraciliochoroidal fluid after trabeculectomy. *Am J Ophthalmol* 1999;**128**:372–5.

Palmberg P, Gonioscopy. Methods of Gonioscopy. In: Ritch R, Shields MB, Krupin T, (eds). The Glaucomas. St Louis: CV Mosby Co, 1996.

Pavlin CJ, Foster FS. Plateau iris syndrome: changes in angle opening associated with dark, light, and pilocarpine administration. *Am J Ophthalmol* 1999;**128**:288–91.

Pavlin CJ, Harasiewicz K, Eng P et al. Ultrasound biomicroscopy of anterior segment structures in normal and glaucomatous eyes. *Am J Ophthalmol* 1992;**113**:381–9.

Pavlin CJ, Harasiewicz K, Foster FS. Posterior iris bowing in pigmentary dispersion syndrome caused by accommodation. *Am J Ophthalmol* 1994;**118**:114–16.

Pavlin CJ, Harasiewicz K, Sherar MD et al. Clinical use of ultrasound biomicroscopy. *Ophthalmology* 1991;**98**:287–95.

Pavlin CJ, McWhae JA, McGowan HD et al. Ultrasound biomicroscopy of anterior segment tumors. *Ophthalmology* 1992;**99**:1220–8.

Pavlin CJ, Ritch R, Foster FS. Ultrasound biomicroscopy in plateau iris syndrome. *Am J Ophthalmol* 1992;**113**:390–5.

Pavlin CJ, Sherar MD, Foster FS. Subsurface ultrasound microscopic imaging of the intact eye. *Ophthalmology* 1990;**97**:244–50.

Potash SD, Tello C, Liebmann J et al. Ultrasound biomicroscopy in pigment dispersion syndrome. *Ophthalmology* 1994;**101**:332–9.

Ritch R. Angle-closure glaucoma. Treatment overview. In: Ritch R, Shields MB, Krupin T, eds. The Glaucomas. St Louis: CV Mosby Co, 1996.

Ritch R, Liebmann J, Tello C. A construct for understanding angle-closure glaucoma: role of ultrasound biomicroscopy. *Ophthalmol Clin N Am* 1995;**8**:281–93.

Shaffer RN. The role of vitreous detachment in aphakic and malignant glaucoma. *Trans Am Acad Ophthalmol Otol* 1954;**58**:217.

Spaeth GL. The normal development of the human chamber angle: a new system of descriptive grading. *Trans Ophthalmol Soc UK* 1971;**91**:709.

Spaeth GL, Aruajo S, Azuara A. Comparison of the configuration of the human anterior chamber angle, as determined by the Spaeth gonioscopic grading system and ultrasound biomicroscopy. *Trans Am Ophthalmol Soc* 1995;**93**:337–47.

Stegman Z, Sokol J, Liebmann JM et al. Reduced trabecular meshwork height in juvenile primary open-angle glaucoma. *Arch Ophthalmol* 1996;**114**:660–3.

Tello C, Liebmann J, Potash SD et al. Measurement of ultrasound biomicroscopy images: intraobserver and interobserver reliaility. *Invest Ophthalmol Vis Sci* 1994;**35**:3549–53.

Tello C, Potash S, Liebmann J et al. Soft contact lens modification of the ocular cup for high resolution ultrasound biomicroscopy. *Ophthalmic Surg* 1994;**24**:563–4.

Urbak SF. Ultrasound biomicroscopy. I. Precision of measurements. *Acta Ophthalmol Scand* 1998;**76**:447–55.

Urbak SF, Pedersen JK, Thorsen TT. Ultrasound biomicroscopy. II. Intraobserver and interobserver reproducibility of measurements. *Acta Ophthalmol Scand* 1998;**76**:546–9.

Wand M, Grant WM, Simmons RJ, Hutchinson BT. Plateau iris syndrome. *Trans Am Acad Ophthalmol Otolaryngol* 1977;**83**:122–30.

5. OPTIC NERVE AND RETINAL NERVE FIBER LAYER

Vital P Costa, Richard P Wilson, and Augusto Azuara-Blanco

Glaucomatous changes in the optic disc

As suggested by George Spaeth, glaucoma is a disease of change. Specifically, change in the appearance of the optic disc is the most important characteristic of the glaucomatous process. Hence, the ability to recognize glaucomatous changes in the optic nerve is fundamental to properly diagnose and manage patients considered suspect for glaucoma or known to have glaucoma (Figure 5.1). The optic

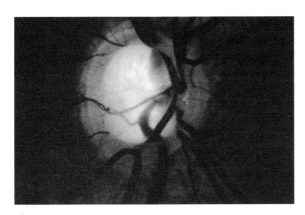

(A)

Figure 5.1A and 5.1B Example of concentric enlargement of the optic nerve cup. The pictures were taken 2 years apart. Observe that both the inferior and superior rims have lost tissue.

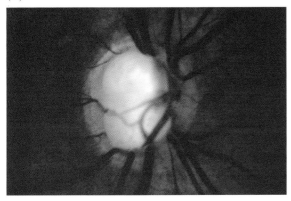

(B)

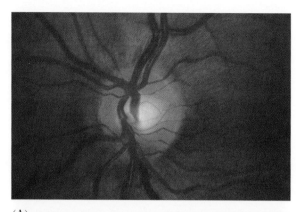

(A)

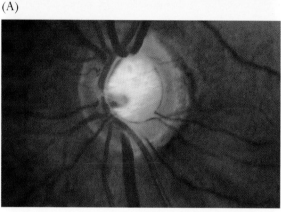

(B)

Figure 5.2
Example of a normal optic disc, following the ISN'T rule: the neural rim is widest in the inferior quadrant, followed by the superior, nasal, and temporal rim (A). Vertical enlargement (B). The superior rim is thinner than the nasal rim, which is against the ISN'T rule.

nerve is damaged by glaucoma in a variety of ways, but irrespective of the pattern of optic nerve damage, it always precedes the development of visual field loss. Thus, the diagnosis of early glaucomatous damage depends on a careful examination of the optic disc and the nerve fiber layer.

In the normal eye, the cup shape is round or horizontally oval, whereas the neural rim is widest in the inferior quadrant, followed by the superior, nasal, and temporal rim (ISN'T rule, see Chapter 1). The mnemonic ISN'T rule appears to be independent of disc size, and in eyes that do not follow this rule glaucoma should be suspected (Figure 5.2).

There are four major patterns of glaucomatous damage to the optic nerve: 1) concentric enlargement of the cup; 2) notching; 3) development of an acquired pit; and 4) development of pallor. In any patient with glaucoma, one or more of these four patterns is usually present.

Although concentric enlargement of the cup is the most common way by which a disc becomes cupped in association with high IOPs, a large cup is not a specific

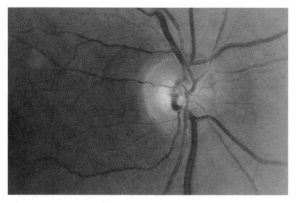

Figure 5.3A and 5.3B Disc asymmetry. Observe that the left eye has a larger cup due to a severe thinning of the inferior rim.

(A)

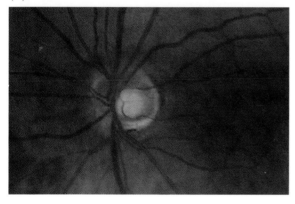

(B)

finding for glaucoma. As previously described, there is a correlation between the optic disc and the optic cup sizes: the larger the optic disc, the larger is the optic cup. This leads to an important clinical guideline: large discs may be associated with physiologically large cups that can appear glaucomatous. On the other hand, apparently normal cups in small discs may already be a sign of glaucomatous damage.

As mentioned previously, the detection of change is diagnostic of glaucomatous damage. Concentric enlargement is characterized by a generalized loss of rim, so that it becomes thinner in all areas (Figure 5.1). Not only can high IOPs lead to concentric enlargement of the cup, but also an acute IOP reduction may result in reversal of cupping.

Temporal unfolding and vertical enlargement are subsets of concentric enlargement of the cup (Figure 5.2B), where the enlargement occurs away from the nasal blood vessels and toward the temporal sector of the disc or vertically.

The presence of asymmetry between the two eyes is also highly suggestive of glaucoma (Figure 5.3). Several studies have shown that cup/disc asymmetries

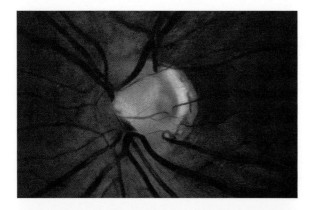

Figure 5.4 Congenital optic nerve pit. Observe that the posterior displacement of the lamina cribrosa occurs at the temporal margin of the disc.

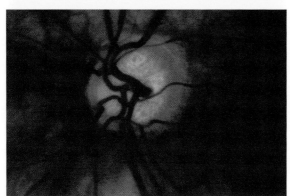

Figure 5.5 Nasal cupping, characterized by loss of tissue in the nasal rim, creating a space between the central vessels and the rim.

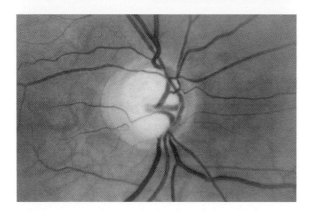

Figure 5.6 Superior baring of the superior circumlinear vessel.

higher than 0.2 are present in less than 1% of the normal population. One has to be careful, however, to exclude other causes for cup/disc asymmetries, such as anisometropia (which can be associated with optic disc asymmetry), myopia, and disc anomalies such as coloboma, congenital pit (Figure 5.4), hypoplasia, and the 'Morning Glory' syndrome.

The extension of the cup toward the nasal side of the optic disc results in another important sign of glaucomatous damage: nasal cupping. In this case, the main blood vessels, which normally lie on the nasal neuroretinal rim, appear separated from the rim by an extension of the cup (normally absent in that area, Figure 5.5). An early sign of neuroretinal rim loss is the baring of a circumlinear vessel, a small arteriole or vein that lies superficially on the superior or inferior neuroretinal rim and leaves the disc toward the macula. As the rim narrows, a space between the rim and the vessel appears (Figure 5.6).

The development of notching, a localized rim loss that may extend to the disc margin, is a highly specific finding for glaucoma. It usually starts at the inner surface of the neuroretinal rim and extends peripherally and posteriorly. Different from the concentric enlargement of the cup, the presence of a notch is frequently associated with a visual field defect (Figures 5.7, 5.8).

The acquired pit of the optic nerve (APON) is another example of localized tissue loss caused by glaucomatous damage that is thought to be almost pathognomonic for glaucoma. It is characterized by a localized loss of optic nerve tissue extending deep into the lamina and to the disc margin (Figure 5.9). It differs from a notch because the latter does not extend deep into the lamina, and does not give the impression of a focal laminar insufficiency. It also differs from congenital optic nerve pits (Figure 5.4). APONs tend to develop at the temporal side of the inferior pole of the optic disc, although about one third may develop next to the superior pole. On the other hand, congenital pits normally appear in the temporal margin of the optic disc, and may be associated with a retinal detachment that can extend to the macular area.

Overpass cupping may be the earliest consistently recognizable sign of early optic nerve damage (Figure 5.10). While it can be seen with optic atrophy of neurological origin, it is usually indicative of glaucoma. In early glaucoma, the initial finding may be increased translucency of the optic nerve centrally. The translucency gradually becomes transparency as the superficial optic nerve tissue atrophies. As the more solid optic nerve tissue recedes posteriorly, the vessels that rested on the surface of the nerve remain in place, supported by the internal limiting membrane of Elschnig. When observed stereoscopically with good magnification and controllable illumination, the vessels appear to bridge over the nerve tissue like an overpass over a road.

Senile sclerosis is a type of glaucomatous damage characterized by shallow and broad cups, associated with peripapillary changes and more marked pallor than would be expected from the amount of cupping. It is common in elderly patients with normal tension glaucoma.

In addition to the previous characteristics, optic disc examination must assess the pallor of the neuroretinal rim. Schwartz has emphasized the importance of pallor in detecting glaucomatous change, but its value may be limited by the subjectivity in judging its intensity, which is influenced by the method

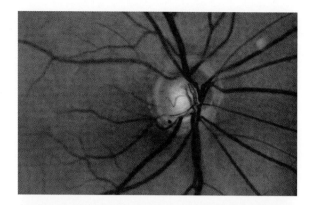

Figure 5.7
Notching. Note a complete loss of neuroretinal rim in the infero-temporal area.

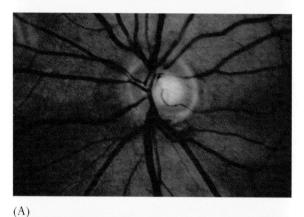

(A)

Figure 5.8A and 5.8B Example of focal progression of optic nerve damage. The pictures were taken 1 year apart. Observe that the inferior rim (already damaged) showed further thinning, displacing the vessel posteriorly.

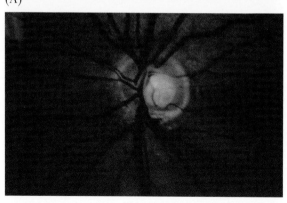

(B)

of examination and the presence of lenticular opacities. Nevertheless, the identification of focal pallor or asymmetric pallor between two eyes may show glaucomatous damage.

Although peripapillary atrophy may be present in non-glaucomatous eyes, there is evidence suggesting that it is more common in eyes with glaucoma.

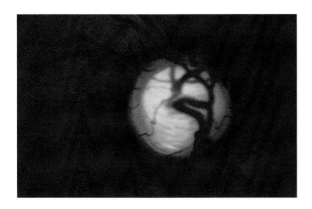

Figure 5.9:
Acquired pit of the optic nerve. Observe that the inferior rim is absent and that there is a localized, posterior displacement of the lamina cribrosa.

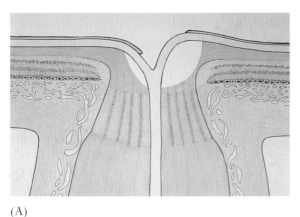

(A)

(B)

Figure 5.10
Overpass cupping is an important early sign of glaucoma. As the superficial neural tissue is lost, the remaining solid optic nerve tissue recedes posteriorly, and the vessels remain in place, supported by the internal limiting membrane of Elschnig. The vessels appear to bridge over the nerve tissue like an overpass over a road (A). With progression of glaucomatous damage, the vessels eventually are displaced posteriorly, and the overpass sign is lost (B). Fig. 5.10 Reproduced with permission from Heilman K, Richardson K. Glaucoma: Conceptions of a Disease. Saunders, 1978 (Figs. 3.33a1, b1–3.33a4, b4).

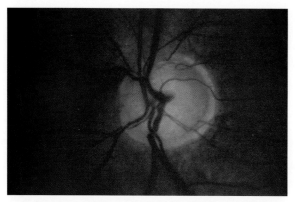

Figure 5.11
Peripapillary atrophy
types alpha
(temporal region),
and beta (inferior
region).

(A)

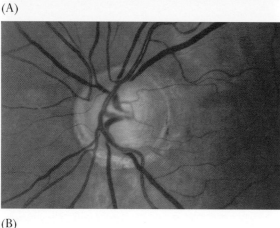

(B)

Peripapillary atrophy can be classified in two zones. The peripheral zone (zone alpha) is characterized by an irregular hypopigmentation and hyperpigmentation with thinning of the chorioretinal tissue. The inner zone (zone beta) is characterized by visible sclera and large choroidal vessels, suggesting a marked atrophy of the chorioretinal tissues, including the retinal pigment epithelium. In glaucomatous eyes, both zones are larger and zone beta is more frequently present than in normals. Moreover, the localization of peripapillary atrophy zone beta has been linked to the visual field defect, and is associated with higher risk of progressive visual field loss (Figure 5.11).

The presence of optic disc hemorrhage has been associated with glaucoma for a long time. The prevalence of optic disc hemorrhages has been estimated at 0 to 0.21% in the normal population and 2.2 to 4.1% in glaucomatous eyes. Disc hemorrhages are small and lie radially near the edge of the disc, most frequently on the inferior rim. They not only represent a sign of glaucomatous damage, but also indicate inadequate control when observed in a patient already known to have glaucoma (Figure 5.12).

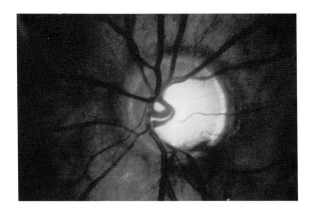

Figure 5.12 Disc hemorrhage in the infero-temporal rim (already damaged).

Examination and documentation of the optic disc

Direct ophthalmoscopy

The assessment of a disc with a direct ophthalmoscope can provide useful information for the diagnosis and management of glaucoma. Direct ophthalmoscopy is best done with the pupils dilated and the room darkened, and with both the examiner and the patient comfortable. The patient should be seated, looking steadily at a fixation target at the same level as the head. The examiner's head also needs to be at the same level as the patient's, without obstructing the fixating eye.

The dioptric power of the ophthalmoscope is set at the spherical equivalent of the patient's refractive error. The illuminating beam needs to be sharply focused on the retina, and the diameter of the beam should be smaller than the width of the optic disc. The opthalmoscope is then moved in order to change the direction of the light entering the pupil, creating shadows that will help to analyse the features of the disc surface and to define the neuroretinal rim. Special attention has to be given to the disc color, its texture, the width of the neuroretinal rim, the cup, and the position of the blood vessels.

The main disadvantage of analysing the disc with the direct ophthalmoscope is the absence of a stereoscopic view. The examiner has to use indirect tips to allow the interpretation of the disc as a three-dimensional structure. Furthermore, direct ophthalmoscopy does not yield a permanent record, and the examiner is required to draw the disc to allow subsequent comparisons.

Binocular ophthalmoscopic techniques

Binocular systems provide the advantage of stereopsis, allowing a three-dimensional observation of the optic disc. However, the indirect ophthalmoscope using a binocular headset with a 20D lens is not a good instrument for this purpose, the limitation being the small magnification of the image, reducing the chances of detection of subtle changes in the optic disc.

A valid option (preferred by the authors) is a standard slit-lamp biomicroscope associated with non-contact lenses (60D or 78D; 90D lenses do not give adequate magnification). As with any indirect opthalmoscopy system, this technique provides an inverted and reversed image of the optic disc, but the magnification is significantly higher than that obtained with the headset. The possibility of stereopsis depends on the pupil's size, which needs to be dilated. The patient is positioned at the slit-lamp and asked to look to the examiner's opposite ear. The examiner views the patient's eye through the slit lamp and then positions the objective lens in the line of sight, about 10–15 mm away from the patient's cornea (Figure 5.•). The fundus image is then brought into sharp focus by slow back-and-forth movements of the biomicroscope.

It is also possible to use the slit lamp in association with a contact lens (e.g. the Goldmann lens), but this technique requires the use of a topical anesthetic and a viscoelastic substance between the lens and the cornea. Despite being more uncomfortable, the image provided is excellent with high magnification, and it is not inverted. Both the contact lens and the Hruby lens allow the use of an off-axis slit beam, which can be focused to accentuate an observer's appreciation of the depth and contour of the cup.

The Hruby lens is a –55D lens, usually attached to the slit lamp, which can be used to examine the optic disc. The lens has to be positioned a few millimeters away from the patient's cornea, and provides a virtual (non-inverted) image, with excellent magnification but a limited field of view. The lens has the advantage of freeing the observer's hand, allowing simultaneous drawing of the disc. However, wide pupils and a steady fixation by the patient are needed. Since the direction of gaze of the observed eye is controlled by fixation of the contralateral eye on the target light, the Hruby lens cannot be used in one-eyed patients.

Drawing the optic disc

The examination of the optic disc needs to be accompanied by documentation of the exam, to allow comparisons and permit the detection of changes that ultimately characterize progression of the disease. Simply describing the cup/disc ratio is a poor, unreliable method, but it continues to be widely used and needs to be discouraged. Completely different discs can be described with the same cup/disc ratio. A disc drawing offers a more detailed way to describe all the features that are important to characterize glaucoma, but there are obvious limitations.

The drawing is subjective and depends on the ability of the examiner to draw. Observers tend to assess the optic disc in different ways, which limits the usefulness of drawings when several ophthalmologists are involved in a patient's care (interobserver variability). Even a single ophthalmologist may do different drawings of a patient with stable glaucoma (intraobserver variability).

Despite these limitations, disc drawings remain a viable, quick, and inexpensive method of monitoring the optic disc in glaucomatous patients. It becomes imperative when other techniques cannot be used owing to limited resources, miotic pupils, or hazy media.

Optic disc photographs

A wide variety of cameras and films are available to provide good, stereoscopic, color pictures of the optic disc. Stereoscopic pictures can be obtained with sequential photographs using a monocular camera by horizontal realignment of the camera base when photographing the same retinal image. The use of +10D lenses and a negatoscope allow the examiner to view the optic disc stereoscopically. Alternatively, simultaneous stereoscopic fundus photographs can be obtained with special cameras that capture two images of the fundus taken simultaneously at a fixed angle between each other (Figure 5.13). These photographs are better than those obtained with sequential pictures because they provide a standard, reproducible view of the optic disc with excellent stereopsis.

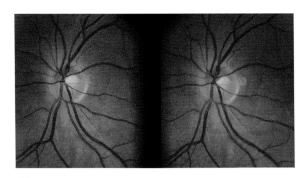

Figure 5.13
Simultaneous stereoscopic fundus photographs of a normal (A) and a glaucomatous eye (B).

(A)

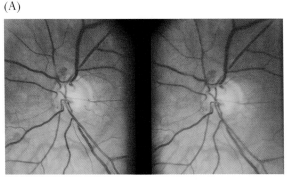

(B)

Stereoscopic slides require development, which precludes the comparison of images obtained that day. By contrast, Polaroid photography provides an instant image that can be viewed by the patient during examination, improving his/her understanding of the disease.

It is important to emphasize, however, that interpretation of stereoscopic photography of the disc varies. In fact, several studies showed that, although interobserver and intraobserver variabilities in estimating cup/disc ratios are higher with a monoscopic view than with a stereoscopic view, the latter is still associated with some interobserver variability in assessing cup/disc ratios and in assessing whether a disc is glaucomatous or not.

Glaucomatous changes in the retinal nerve fiber layer

The retinal nerve fiber layer is formed by about 1.2 million ganglion cell axons. The axons of the ganglion cells nasal to the optic disc run directly toward the optic disc, similarly to the axons originated in the macular area that form the papillomacular bundle. The axons coming from ganglion cells situated in the temporal fundus describe an arc around the fovea and run toward the superior or inferior poles of the optic disc (see Chapter 1). The nerve fiber layer is thickest at the vertical optic disc poles and thinner at the temporal and nasal optic disc borders. This pattern can be observed in black and white, red-free, wide-angle fundus photographs, which show the nerve fiber bundles as bright striations in the retinal reflex (Figure 5.14).

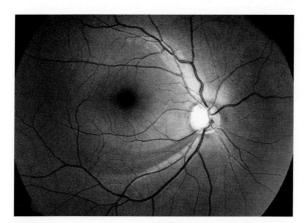

Figure 5.14 Nerve fiber layer defects. Black-and-white nerve fiber layer photograph showing a typical defect in the inferior bundle compatible with glaucomatous optic nerve damage. Fig 5.14 Reproduced with permission from Gamero GE, Fechtner RD. The optic nerve in glaucoma. In: Choplin NT, Lundy DC, eds. Atlas of Glaucoma. London; Martin Dunitz, 1998).

In 1987, Hoyt and Newman first described retinal nerve fiber layer (RNFL) defects as an early sign of glaucoma. Subsequently, several studies confirmed the importance of RNFL assessment in the diagnosis and management of glaucoma. Sommer and colleagues have shown that RNFL abnormalities are one of the first clinically detectable changes in patients with glaucoma, and may precede visual field damage by up to 5 years. Histological studies support these findings and suggest that a 40% loss of nerve fibers is possible in the presence of a normal Goldmann visual field examination.

RNFL defects may be localized (wedge and slit defects), or diffuse. Slit-like or groove-like defects are judged a sign of abnormality when they extend to the disc margin. In some eyes, localized, wedge-shaped defects in the RNFL can be seen in the superior or inferior arcuate areas, normally associated with notches in the neuroretinal rim. They are visualized as dark areas without striations, by contrast to the adjacent normal RNFL (Figure 5.14). Although localized defects are easier to detect, diffuse RNFL loss is more common and more difficult to diagnose. It is characterized by the visualization of second order retinal vessels, which are normally invisible and hidden by the RNFL. As the glaucomatous damage increases, there is a progressive loss of the RNFL in both the superior and inferior poles, but the RNFL in the papillomacular bundle remains intact. In end-stage glaucoma, no striations are found, and a diffuse RNFL loss is observed.

The RNFL may be examined through a dilated pupil, with a red-free light and a direct ophthalmoscope. However, a better view can be obtained with a 78D or 90D lens or a contact lens at the slit lamp with a green filter. Slit lamp examination allows the detection of localized RNFL loss, depending on the examiner's experience. Alternatively, the RNFL may be documented using high resolution black and white pictures, in which the fiber bundles are seen as silver striations most visible in the superior and inferior poles of the optic disc. This method was first introduced by Behrendt and Wilson, and was subsequently improved by other authors.

The technique includes the use of a green or blue filter, a high-contrast, fine-grain, black and white film, and a special development method. However, the results of black and white photography of the RNFL are limited in eyes with small pupils and media opacities. Furthermore, the technique is subjective and depends on the examiner's experience: inexperienced examiners tend to overestimate localized defects and underestimate diffuse RNFL loss. Semiquantitative RNFL scores have been developed, but they still rely on subjective criteria and depend on the examiner's experience.

Quantitative measurements of the optic disc and retinal nerve fiber layer

Devices that allow quantitative measurements of the optic nerve and the retinal nerve fiber layer were developed to reduce intra- and interobserver variability, providing reproducible, objective data either to diagnose or to monitor the progression of optic disc/RNFL damage. The first quantitative techniques used stereophotographs as a working tool.

Planimetry includes the determination of the disc rim and disc edge by tracing projected images while viewing a corresponding stereoscopic pair. A computerized planimeter is then used to measure the disc area, a measurement that has been used to analyse progression in prospective studies. Photogrammetry, on the other hand, uses stereophotographs to allow three-dimensional measurements of the optic disc topography. These techniques require the observer to trace the edge of the disc and cup, are time-consuming, and are subject to some degree of variability.

Computerized image analysis has been used to allow quantitative measurements, initially via digitized, simultaneous, stereoscopic, videographic images. These instruments included the Topcon Imagenet (Figure 5.15) and the Rodenstock Optic Nerve Analyzer (Rodenstock Instruments, Munich, Germany), which were limited by the suboptimal resolution of images and poor reproducibility. Confocal laser scanning imaging technology, used by the Heidelberg Retina Tomograph (Heidelberg Engineering, Heidelberg, Germany) and the

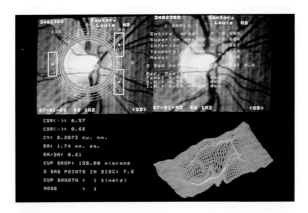

Figure 5.15 Optic nerve topography obtained with the Imagenet (Topcon).

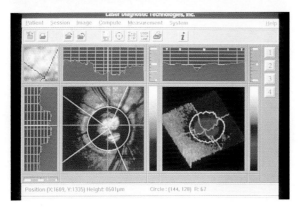

Figure 5.16 Optic nerve topography obtained with a confocal scanning laser ophthalmoscope (TOPSS, Laser Diagnostic Technologies, San Diego, USA).

TOPSS (Laser Diagnostic Technologies, San Diego, USA) (Figure 5.16), does not require pupil dilation and exploits the principle of confocal laser scanning to allow quantitative structural information (Figure 5.17) with high resolution and good

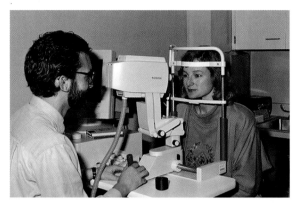

(A)

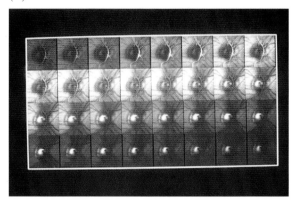

(B)

Figure 5.17
Acquisition of optic disc images with a confocal scanning laser ophthalmoscope (Heidelberg Retina Tomograph, HRT, Heidelberg Instruments, Heidelberg, Germany), (A). A total of 32 evenly spaced consecutive corneal sections of the optic nerve head are obtained, from the most superficial anterior surface to the posteriormost plane just below the bottom of the cup (B). Three-dimensional representation of the optic disc topography as evaluated by the HRT (C).

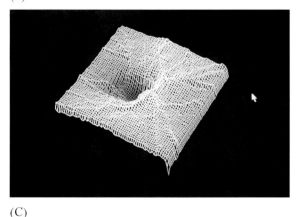

(C)

continued overleaf

63

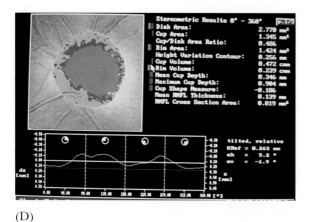

Figure 5.17
continued Example of data output from the HRT: measurements quantifying the disc, rim, cup, cup shape, and retinal nerve fiber layer contour are displayed (D).

(D)

reproducibility. These systems can take several measurements of the optic disc topography, including neural rim and cup area, volume, and shape of the cup contour.

Scanning Laser Polarimetry (GDx, Laser Diagnostic Technologies, San Diego, USA) measures the RNFL thickness. It is based on the birefringent properties of the RNFL, which has its neurotubules disposed in an organized, parallel fashion. This peculiar anatomy leads to a change in the state of polarized light as it passes through the RNFL, slowing the light in direct proportion to its thickness. Experimental and clinical studies have shown that SLP provides quantitative and reproducible measurements of the RNFL (Figure 5.18).

The RNFL thickness can also be assessed through Optical Coherence Tomography (OCT), an optical analog of B-scan ultrasound that can create high-resolution cross-sectional images of the RNFL.

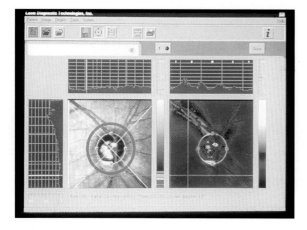

Figure 5.18
Scanning laser polarimetry (GDx, Laser Diagnostic Technologies, San Diego, USA). Red signals show areas with greater retardation and nerve fiber layer thickness.

Irrespective of the instrument, it is important to emphasize that, although these technologies seem promising, optic disc topography and RNFL thickness among the general population are highly variable, which limits their use in the detection of early glaucoma. At present, they cannot replace an experienced examiner. Longitudinal studies are being done to determine the ability of these systems to detect changes in the optic disc or RNFL, indicating what can be considered a true sign of progression in glaucomatous patients. The increasing use of image analysers in research and office settings, and the introduction of modifications specifically designed to neutralize their limitations, will increase their role in clinical practice.

Suggested reading

Airaksinen PJ, Tuulonen A, Werner EB. Clinical evaluation of the optic disc and retinal nerve fiber layer. In: Ritch R, Shields MB, Krupin T (eds). *The Glaucomas*, 2nd edition. St Louis M.: CV Mosby Co, 1996; 617–57.

Drance SM, Fairclough M, Butler DM, Kottler MS. The importance of disc hemorrhage in the prognosis of chronic open angle glaucoma. *Arch Ophthalmol* 1977; **95**:226–8.

Hitchings RA, Spaeth GL. The optic disc in glaucoma. I. Classification. *Br J Ophthalmol* 1976;**60**:778–85.

Jonas JB, Fernandez MC, Naumann GOH. Glaucomatous parapapillary atrophy. Occurrence and correlations. *Arch Ophthalmol* 1992;**110**:214–222.

Lichter PR. Variability of expert observers in evaluating the optic disc. *Trans Am Ophthalmol Soc* 1976;**74**:532–72.

Mikelberg FS, Drance SM, Schulzer M et al. The normal human optic nerve. *Ophthalmology* 1989;**96**:1325–8.

Osher RH, Herschler J. The significance of baring of the circumlinear vessel: a prospective study. *Arch Ophthalmol* 1981;**99**:817–8.

Pederson JE, Anderson DR. The mode of progressive disc cupping in ocular hypertension and glaucoma. *Arch Ophthalmol* 1980;**98**:490–5.

Quigley HA, Addicks EM, Green WR. Optic nerve damage in human glaucoma. III. Quantitative correlation of nerve fiber loss and visual field defect in glaucoma, ischemic neuropathy, papilledema, and toxic neuropathy. *Arch Ophthalmol* 1982;**100**:135–46.

Quigley HA, Addicks EM. Regional differences in the structure of the lamina cribrosa and their relation to glaucomatous optic nerve damage. *Arch Ophthalmol* 1981;**99**:137–43.

Sharma NK, Hitchings RA. A comparison of monocular and stereoscopic photographs of the optic disc in the identification of glaucomatous visual field defects. *Br J Ophthalmol* 1983;**67**:677–80.

Sommer A, Katz J, Quigley HA et al. Clinically detectable nerve fiber atrophy precedes the onset of glaucomatous field loss. *Arch Ophthalmol* 1991;**109**:77–83.

Spaeth GL, Hitchings RA. The optic disc in glaucoma: pathogenic correlation of five patterns of cupping in chronic open angle glaucoma. *Trans Am Acad Ophthalmol Otolaryngol* 1976; **81**:217–23.

Varma R, Spaeth GL. *The optic nerve in glaucoma.* Philadelphia, PA: Lippincott, 1993.

Varma R, Steinmann WC, Scott IU. Expert agreement in evaluating the optic disc for glaucoma. *Ophthalmology* 1992;**99**:215–22.

Weinreb RN, Shakiba S, Zangwill L. Scanning laser polarimetry to measure the nerve fiber layer of normal and glaucomatous eyes. *Am J Ophthalmol* 1994;**119**:627–36.

6. Visual Field and Other Functional Tests in Glaucoma

Vital P Costa, Richard P Wilson, and Augusto Azuara-Blanco

Visual field and other functional tests

Visual field

Definition and characteristics

The visual field can be defined as the portion of space in which objects can be simultaneously seen when the eye is looking in one fixed direction. In other words, when looking at an object, the group of images perceived by the eye at a given instant is called the visual field.

The monocular visual field has an elliptical format, extending 60 degrees superiorly, 75 degrees inferiorly, 60–65 degrees nasally, and 100–110 degrees temporally. The binocular visual field extends about 180 degrees across the horizontal meridian. The central 120 degrees can be seen simultaneously by both eyes, whereas the peripheral 30 degrees are covered by one eye only. For clinical purposes, testing the monocular visual field is more useful than testing the binocular visual field.

Relation between the retina, the optic disc and the visual field

Every point in the retina matches with an area of the visual field. In the same way as a camera, objects situated in the superior visual field are seen by the inferior retina and vice versa. The nasal retina sees objects in the temporal visual field and vice versa.

The center of the visual field, or the point of fixation, is represented by the fovea. The optic nerve does not have photoreceptors and is a region in the visual field where stimuli cannot be seen. Since the optic nerve is situated nasally and slightly above the fovea, this physiological scotoma or physiological blind spot appears 15–17 degrees from fixation in the temporal visual field, slightly below the horizontal meridian. Because the visual field diagram represents the field as the patient sees it, the blind spot appears to the right of fixation in the right eye and to the left of fixation in the left eye.

Basic concepts

The main purpose of visual field testing is not to determine the outer boundary of the field, but to investigate several locations within the boundary that are preferentially damaged in glaucoma. Instead of testing visual acuity at each of these points, static perimetry tests their *threshold* of visual sensitivity, defined as

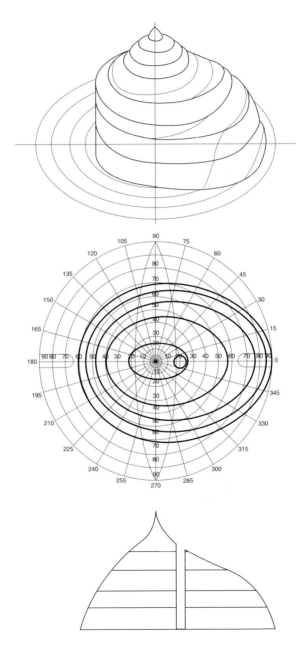

the least intense stimulus perceived by each point. A stimulus that is weaker than the threshold stimulus, and thus is not seen at that point of the visual field, is called an infrathreshold stimulus. Conversely, stimuli that are stronger than the threshold stimulus will always be seen at that particular point and are known as suprathreshold stimuli. When examining the visual field, the term *scotoma* refers to a region where the sensitivity to light is partially (relative scotoma) or totally (absolute scotoma) compromised.

Retinal sensitivity to light is greatest in the fovea, decreasing progressively as it approaches the retinal periphery. This situation has been nicely illustrated by Traquair, who defined the normal visual field as an island of vision surrounded by a sea of blindness (Figure 6.1).

Methods of visual field examination

Confrontation technique

This is a simple technique that investigates the boundaries of the visual field and can be used at the office. The patient is positioned about 1 m away from the examiner, with one eye occluded. The examiner occludes his contralateral eye and asks the patient to fixate at his nose. The examiner presents an object (fingers, bottles) from the periphery toward the center of the visual field until the patient starts noticing it (Figure 6.2). A normal confrontation would show the examiner's visual field coinciding with the patient's. A variation of the

← *Figure 6.1* Characteristics of a normal visual field (right eye) and methods to map it. The visual field is defined as Traquair's 'island of vision surrounded by a sea of blindness'. The top of the figure represents the three-dimensional structure of a normal island of vision. The height of the island of vision (*z-axis*) is highest at its center (fovea). The job of visual field testing is to draw a map of the island of vision. Two different methods are available for drawing a map of the island. The middle of the figure represents the island as viewed from above as drawn by isopter perimetry, such as the Goldmann perimeter. The isopters are determined by moving stimuli from areas of nonseeing towards the center until the patient indicates it has been seen (kinetic perimetry). The bottom of the figure represents a 'slice' or profile of the island of vision through a meridian. It is determined by varying the intensity of a stimulus of fixed size at each point along the meridian until threshold has been determined (static perimetry). Fig 6.1 Reproduced with permission from Choplin NT. Psychophysical and electrophysical testing in glaucoma: visual fields and other functional tests. In: Choplin NT, Lundy DC, eds. Atlas of Glaucoma. London; Martin Dunitz, 1988).

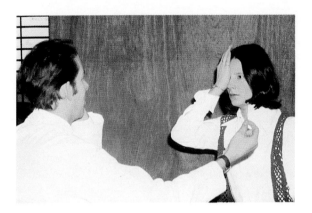

Figure 6.2
Confrontation
technique.

technique investigates the ability of the patient to count fingers in different quadrants. Despite being a subjective, imprecise method, confrontation allows a quick assessment of patients such as children who do not perform well in more objective methods. In some cases, the technique can also be used to confirm unsuspected visual field defects found on perimetry.

Kinetic perimetry

In kinetic perimetry, a stimulus is moved from a region where it is not visible (infrathreshold) to a region where it becomes visible (suprathreshold). The boundary between suprathreshold and infrathreshold regions is called *isopter*—a line that connects points of equal threshold.

The Goldmann perimeter is the most widely used instrument for kinetic perimetry. The size and brightness of the perimetric targets can be varied, which allows the determination of several isopters and investigation of the extension and depth of scotomas. Small isopters near the center represent areas of high retinal sensitivities, defined by low threshold stimuli. Larger isopters in the periphery of the field represent areas of low retinal sensitivities, defined by bright threshold stimuli (Figures 6.1 and 6.3).

Static perimetry

Static perimetry estimates the threshold sensitivity of several points within the visual field. Unlike kinetic perimetry, the target locations remain constant and the brightness is **increased** until the threshold sensitivity is **reached** (Figures 6.1 and 6.3). In theory, both kinetic and static perimetry should give similar results. In practice, moving objects tend to be more visible than stationary ones, especially in defective areas of the field (the Riddoch phenomenon).

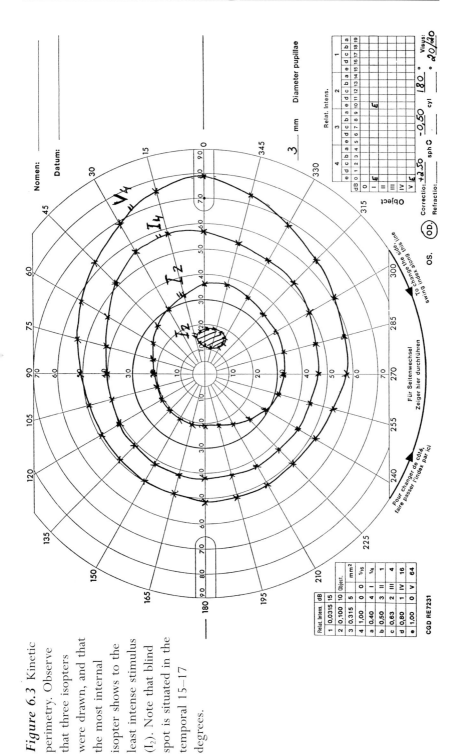

Figure 6.3 Kinetic perimetry. Observe that three isopters were drawn, and that the most internal isopter shows to the least intense stimulus (I_2). Note that blind spot is situated in the temporal 15–17 degrees.

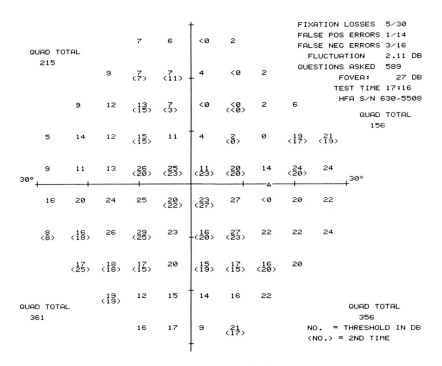

Figure 6.4 Static perimetry of the central 30 degrees. Each number relates to the threshold sensitivity in each point, measured in decibels. Threshold values resulting from repeated determinations are in parenthesis.

Automated or computerized perimetry uses static perimetry and reports its results as threshold sensitivity values printed on a numeric grid (Figure 6.4). The Goldmann perimeter also allows static perimetry to be done. In fact, the preferred method to investigate glaucomatous visual field defects with the Goldmann perimeter, described by Armaly and further modified by Drance, uses both kinetic and static strategies.

Manual vs. automated perimetry

Manual perimetry relies on the examiner's skill and technique, making comparisons between different exams performed in different institutions very difficult. Furthermore, it does not measure short-term fluctuation, does not have catch trials to assess the reliability of the exam, and does not supply a statistical package for comparison with a normal database.

Automated perimetry, on the other hand, uses a standard algorithm to determine the threshold sensitivity of each tested point, reducing the influence of the examiner. Hence, if a patient undergoes visual field examination using the same

72

instrument in different institutions, the ophthalmologist will be better able to compare the different tests. Furthermore, automated perimetry is able to quantify short-term fluctuation, analyse reliability, and compare the actual examination to an age-matched normal database.

Finally, automated perimetry is capable of detecting glaucomatous visual field defects earlier than manual perimetry. For these reasons, automated perimetry, which has become the gold standard in visual field examination of glaucomatous patients, will be focused upon in this chapter.

Visual field loss in glaucoma

Visual field loss in glaucoma is a prechiasmatic defect secondary to the loss of axons that form the optic nerve. To allow a correct interpretation of the visual field in glaucoma, one should remember the anatomic pattern of the retinal nerve fiber layer (RNFL) and its relation with the optic disc (See Chapter 1).

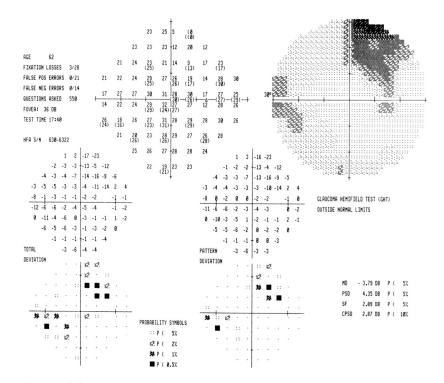

Figure 6.5 Full-threshold Humphrey's superior Seidel scotoma in a patient with early glaucomatous damage. Observe that four contiguous points adjacent to the blind spot have abnormally low sensitivities, the corrected pattern standard deviation index is slightly raised, and the glaucoma hemifield test is outside normal limits.

73

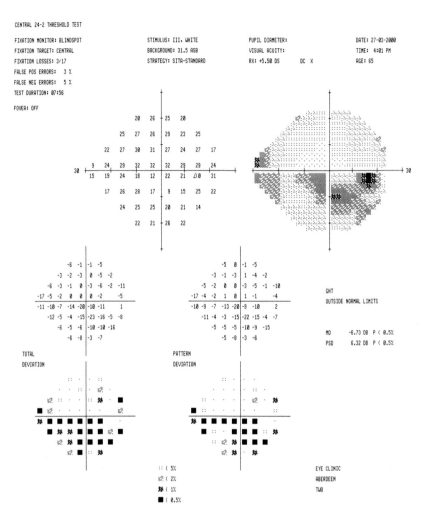

Figure 6.6 Humphrey's SITA 24–2 with an inferior loss involving the arcuate, paracentral and nasal visual field.

In summary, the axons nasal to the optic disc run directly toward the optic disc, similarly to the axons originated in the macular area, which form the papillo-macular bundle. The axons coming from ganglion cells situated in the temporal fundus describe an arcuate course around the fovea and run toward the superior or inferior poles of the optic disc. This explains why an infero-temporal notch in the optic disc relates to a visual field defect in the supero-nasal quadrant.

The first nerve fibers to be damaged in glaucoma are typically the ones entering the superior or inferior poles of the optic disc. Thus, the classic glaucomatous visual field defect begins as scotomas within the area of Bjerrum (Figure 6.5). These scotomas tend to coalesce and progressively

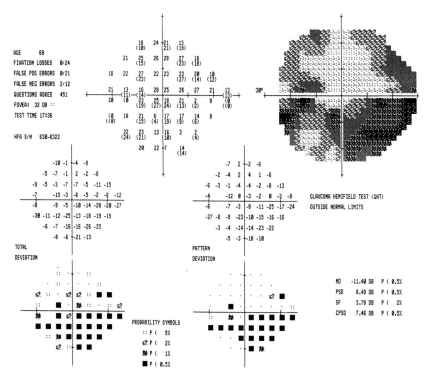

Figure 6.7 Full-threshold Humphrey's 24–2 test with severe loss: inferior arcuate scotoma and nasal step. Note that the corrected pattern standard deviation is significantly raised (7.46 dB, $p < 0.5\%$), and the mean deviation severely reduced (−11.48 dB, $p < 0.5\%$).

occupy the entire Bjerrum area, extending from the nasal periphery to the blind spot and forming a complete arcuate scotoma (Figures 6.6 and 6.7). Nasal steps are common glaucomatous visual field defects and occur when there is a difference in sensitivity above and below the horizontal raphe nasal to fixation (Figure 6.7). The central 10 degrees of the visual field, which correspond to the papillomacular bundle, are usually preserved until late in the course of the disease, providing the patient with a central island of vision and good visual acuity. However, localized paracentral scotomas near fixation may be more common in patients with low tension glaucoma (Chapter 7). The peripheral temporal visual field is also normally preserved, except in rare cases in which a temporal wedge defect occurs with its apex at the blind spot.

Although this is the classic progression of the visual field in glaucoma, the type and the rate of visual field loss in glaucoma are variable. Localized defects in the arcuate area of Bjerrum are characteristic of glaucoma, but uniform, diffuse visual field loss is also possible.

75

Automated perimetry

Computers were first associated with visual field testing in the mid-1970s. Many automated perimeters have been developed since then, but the two most commonly used worldwide are the Octopus perimeter (Interzeag, Switzerland), and the Humphrey perimeter (Humphrey, USA). This chapter will focus on the interpretation of Humphrey's visual field tests, but the principles described below can be applied to any computerized perimeter.

Size and brightness of the stimulus

The Humphrey perimeter uses Goldmann stimulus sizes, varying from I to V. The stimulus size III, with an area of 4 mm^2, is routinely used but may be modified by the examiner. For example, automated perimetry with a size V stimulus may be best in patients with low visual acuity (less than 20/200).

The brightness of the stimulus can be measured with absolute or relative units. An apostilb (asb) is an absolute unit of brightness per unit area, defined as 0.31831 (1/π) candela/m^2. Because the range of thresholds recordable in automated perimetry is very large, varying from less than 1 asb to 10 000 asb, perimetric stimuli are expressed in a relative unit: decibels (dB). One decibel equals 0.1 logarithmic unit of attenuation of the maximum stimulus intensity. Since the maximum stimulus provided by the Humphrey instrument is 10 000 asb, a 10 dB stimulus is obtained after a 1.0 logarithmic unit of attenuation, allowing 10% of the maximum stimulus to be transmitted. On the other hand, a 0 dB stimulus is equivalent to the maximum stimulus. The decibel scale is not standardized among perimeters, since the maximum luminance of the stimulus varies between instruments (e.g. a 20 dB stimulus in the Humphrey perimeter is not equivalent to a 20 dB stimulus in the Octopus perimeter). The result is that decibel values close to zero indicate defective areas of low sensitivity, whereas high numbers characterize normal areas. It is important to note that 0 dB does not necessarily mean a blind area, but rather a location where the sensitivity of the retina is below the maximum brightness presented by the perimeter.

Programs and strategies

In modern Humphrey perimeters, there are four algorithms for determining threshold sensitivity at each test location: Standard Full Threshold, Fastpac, SITA Standard, and SITA Fast. Ideally, testing strategies should be accurate and fast because fatigue (associated with long test times) causes depression of threshold sensitivity, increased defect artifact, and greater variability. The Standard Full Threshold algorithm, which has been used for the past two decades, is accurate

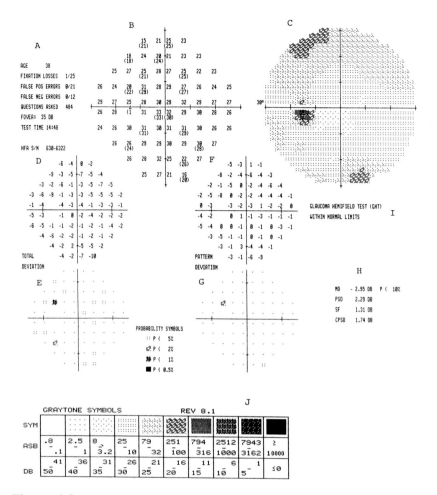

Figure 6.8 Printout of a full-threshold Humphrey's 30–2 program illustrating the reliability indices (A), the numeric grid (B), the grayscale (C), the total deviation numeric (D) and probability (E) plots, the pattern deviation numeric (F) and probability (G) plots, the global indices (H), the glaucoma hemifield test (I), and the graytone scale (J).

but very time consuming (Figure 6.8). Test durations of more than 15 min are common in patients with glaucomatous defects. Shorter tests such as the Fastpac have been designed, but are less sensitive and subject to greater variability. Recently, the SITA strategy has been introduced in Humphrey perimeters, showing the same accuracy as the Full Threshold algorithm with much shorter test times. SITA Fast further reduces testing time. SITA Standard is becoming the procedure of choice for the assessment of visual fields with Humphrey's perimeters. This chapter will concentrate on the Full Threshold and SITA Standard strategies, because they are the most accurate and reliable for evaluating visual fields in glaucoma with Humphrey's visual fields.

Examination of the visual field in glaucoma is usually limited to the central 30-degree area, since almost all clinically relevant defects fall within this area (Figure 6.8). The Central 30-2 test measures the retinal sensitivity at points extending around fixation for 30 degrees in all directions using a size III stimulus. Test points are aligned every 6 degrees of the vertical and horizontal meridians. The Central 24-2 test, which evaluates the temporal 24-degree and nasal

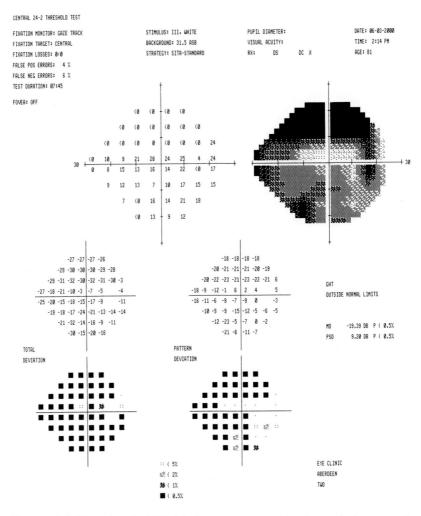

Figure 6.9 Humphrey's SITA 24–2 in a patient with advanced glaucoma. A severe constriction of the visual field is noted.

30-degree area is a widely used alternative, because it reduces the testing time without significantly compromising its ability to detect visual field loss, especially nasal steps (Figure 6.9).

In the Standard Full Threshold algorithm, the sensitivity of each location is determined with a bracketing or staircase strategy. The program initially determines the threshold level at four primary points. If the initial stimulus is seen, its intensity is decreased in 4 dB steps until it is not seen. The intensity is then increased in 2 dB steps until the patient sees the stimulus. Similarly, if the patient does not see the first stimulus, the same process is done in reverse. The value last seen is registered as the threshold of that particular location. The threshold values of the four primary points, situated 9 degrees from the vertical and horizontal medians in each quadrant, are used as the starting test levels for the neighboring points. When the measured threshold for a point departs from the expected value, the location is re-staircased. In addition to the four primary points, six other locations have the thresholding procedure done twice (Figure 6.8). The test–retest difference in sensitivity is used to calculate the intra-test variability or short-term fluctuation (SF, see below).

In the SITA algorithm, threshold values and measurement errors of threshold values are continuously estimated during the test, using maximum posterior probability calculations in the visual field models. Initially, models are based on prior knowledge of visual fields (using a large database of normal and glaucomatous subjects), and are available before the actual test starts. During the test, staircase procedures are used to alter stimulus intensities at predetermined test point locations. Staircases are interrupted when measurement errors have been reduced to a certain level. This novelty is the main reason for the test time reduction. Test time is further reduced by the elimination of catch trials and through the use of a more effective timing algorithm.

Reliability indices

To assess the reliability of the test, 'catch trials' were developed to assess the steadiness of fixation, the incidence of false negative and false positive responses. These indices appear in the upper left-hand portion of the printout (Figures 6.8 and 6.9). The first versions of the Humphrey perimeter used the Heijl-Krakau method of fixation monitoring. The method includes the presentation of stimuli at the expected location of the blind spot, and assumes that, if the patient responds to such stimulus, a gaze error has occurred. The 'gaze monitor', available in recent models, records and charts gaze direction at the time of each stimulus presentation. Deviations of gaze are indicated by upward deflections in the tracing (at the bottom of the printout). When the gaze monitor is available, the blind spot technique does not need to be used. Numerous deflections indicate poor fixation.

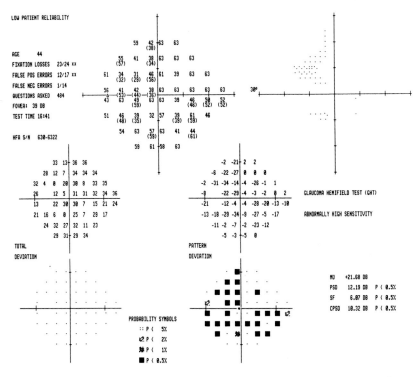

Figure 6.10 Full-threshold Humphrey's 24–2 program in a patient with a high false-positive rate ('trigger happy'). Observe that the grayscale is almost white due to abnormally high sensitivities. This test must be repeated.

False-positive errors occur when the patient responds when no stimulus is presented (Figure 6.10). False-negative trials involve the presentation of supra-threshold stimuli (9 dB more intense) at randomly selected visual field locations where the threshold had been previously determined. If the patient does not respond to this stimulus, a false-negative response is recorded (Figure 6.11). In general, with the Full Threshold algorithm, fixation losses higher than 20%, false-positive or false-negative responses higher than 33% are indicative of an unreliable examination. With SITA, tests with a false-positive or false-negative rates of more than than 15% should be interpreted with caution.

During a visual field examination using the SITA algorithm, catch trials are not done in the same way as described above. In fact, reliability indices are inferred by the SITA algorithm, which helps to reduce the test time.

Numeric grid
This is the first graph appearing in the upper left portion of the printout, below the reliability indices. The numbers represent the measured threshold of each

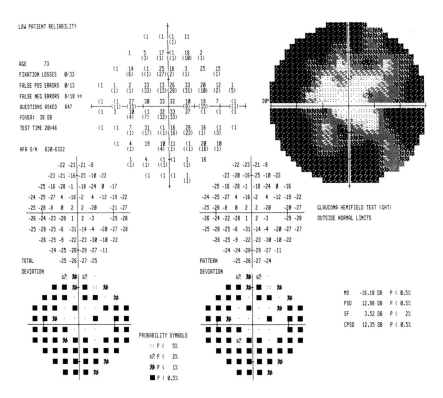

Figure 6.11 Full threshold Humphrey's 30–2 program in a patient with high false-negative rates due to fatigue. Note that the peripheral points (tested at the end of the exam) show poor sensitivities compared to the central points (tested at the beginning of the test), giving a typical cloverleaf pattern. This test must be repeated.

test location. When the Full Threshold algorithm is done, numbers in brackets represent points where the threshold was measured twice, to allow calculation of the short-term fluctuation (Figure 6.8). The SITA algorithm does not measure the short-term fluctuation, and thus does not show numbers in brackets (Figure 6.9).

Grayscale

The grayscale display, situated on the right of the numerical graphic, assigns different shades of gray to different ranges of threshold sensitivity. Areas of lower sensitivity (such as the blind spot) are represented by darker shades, whereas lighter shades indicate higher sensitivities. Although it allows the visualization of defective areas, the grayscale display interpolates values between actual test locations and often hides discrete scotomas.

Total deviation and pattern deviation

In the total deviation graph, the numbers represent the difference between the actual threshold of each test point and the age-corrected normal value for that point. Positive values indicate that the threshold in the actual examination is higher than the expected in the normal population of the same age, whereas negative values show lower sensitivities. In the pattern deviation graph, the numbers represent the total deviation values minus the general height of the hill of vision. The purpose of this adjustment is to highlight localized defects, typical of glaucoma, by removing the effects of generalized loss of sensitivity swing to cataract or small pupil size (Figure 6.12). Below the numerical displays, the probability plots highlight the significance of each measured deviation (e.g. points at which deviations exceed those found in fewer than 5%, 2%, 1%, and

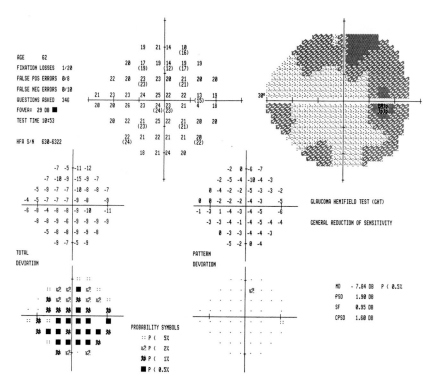

Figure 6.12 Full threshold Humphrey's 24–2 visual field of a 62-year-old patient with cataract in the right eye (visual acuity OD = 20/200). Observe that there is an overall depression characterized by a decreased foveal threshold (29 dB), a significantly reduced mean deviation (−7.84 dB), several points with *p* < 0.5% in the total deviation probability plot and a normal pattern deviation probability plot. Note that the glaucoma hemifield test indicates general reduction of sensitivity.

82

0.5% of normal subjects). The key to the representation of the probability symbols is shown near the bottom of the printout. The symbols increase in darkness as the deviation becomes more significant.

Global Indices

The global indices, displayed in the lower right corner of the printout, are derived from statistical treatment of the raw data to help summarize the information of all measured thresholds.

MD stands for mean deviation and represents the weighted average of the total deviation values. The values near the center receive more weight than those in the periphery. MD is a reflection of the general sensitivity of the field: it is close to zero in a normal examination, and negative when the sensitivity is reduced.

Pattern standard deviation (PSD) is a measure of the variability of the hill of vision, and is high whenever a localized defect is observed.

Short-term fluctuation (SF) measures the intratest variability, and is estimated from duplicate measurements at some locations. It is abnormally high in patients who do not perform well during the test due to fatigue or poor attentiveness. SF is used in combination with the PSD to calculate the corrected pattern standard deviation (CPSD), an index that attempts to remove the variability from the PSD that the patient showed while taking the test, revealing just the irregularity of the visual field due to pathological loss (Figure 6.8). Since the SITA algorithm does not perform duplicate measurements of threshold, its printout does not include the SF and CPSD (Figure 6.9). If any of the global indices fall outside the normal range, they are followed by a probability value ($p < 10\%$, $p < 5\%$, $p < 2\%$, $p < 1\%$, or $p < 0.5\%$).

Glaucoma hemifield test

The visual field damage in glaucoma is frequently asymmetrical, with one of the hemispheres being damaged before the other. Hence, the glaucoma hemifield test (GHT) compares five areas of the superior and inferior hemifields (Figure 6.13). It is available in the 24-2 and 30-2 tests, and its result appears above the global indices. When at least one pair of areas shows a difference that exceeds that found in 99% of the normal population, an *'outside normal limits'* message is displayed. When this difference exceeds that found in 97% of the normal population, a *'borderline'* message is displayed. *'General reduction of sensitivity'* appears when the general height is depressed to a level observed in less than 0.5% of the normal population, whereas *'abnormally high sensitivity'* appears when the general height is higher than that found in 99.5% of the normal population. When none of the above conditions are met, the GHT is considered to be *'within normal limits'*.

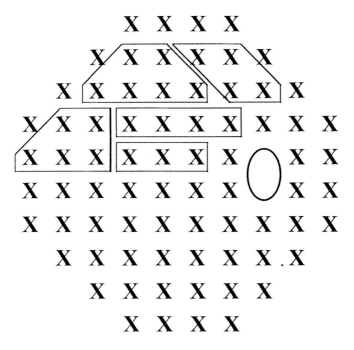

Figure 6.13 Graphic illustration of the five zones analysed in the glaucoma hemifield test (superior hemifield).

Interpreting the visual field

An automated perimetry printout presents an intimidating combination of numbers, graphs, and indices. The examiner needs to understand the meaning of each graph and index in order to interpret the available information correctly. Initially, there are some general guidelines that need to be followed:

a) A normal visual field does not exclude the presence of glaucoma (since visual field defects appear late in the disease), and a typical nerve fiber bundle defect is not necessarily indicative of glaucoma since other conditions such as optic disc drusen, branch retinal vein occlusion, or other optic nerve or chorio-retinal lesions may result in a similar defect (Figure 6.14).

b) The first visual field examination should be interpreted with caution. A learning effect is expected, and some patients may require two or more fields before a reliable examination can be made.

c) To characterize a localized visual field defect, two conditions need to be fulfilled: the defect should affect three or more adjacent and non-peripheral

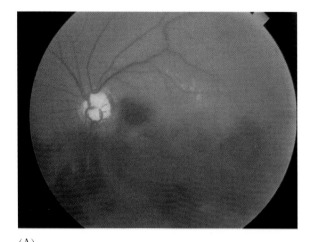

(A)

Figure 6.14A and 6.14B Fundus photograph and visual field of a patient with an inferior hemispheric retinal vein occlusion. The visual field shows a superior field loss, undistinguishable from one caused by advanced glaucomatous damage.

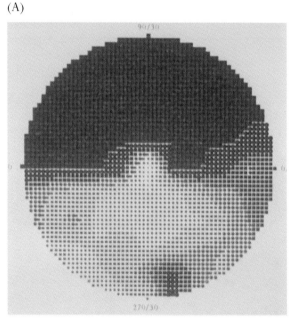

(B)

points in the pattern deviation plot, and it needs to be confirmed by subsequent examinations (Figure 6.15).

d) The same principles apply to the diagnosis of progression. Some degree of change in threshold sensitivity is expected between one examination and another due to long-term fluctuation (Figures 6.16 and 6.17).

e) Visual fields should be interpreted in association with the clinical information. As a subsidiary examination, it should not be evaluated as an independent tool.

85

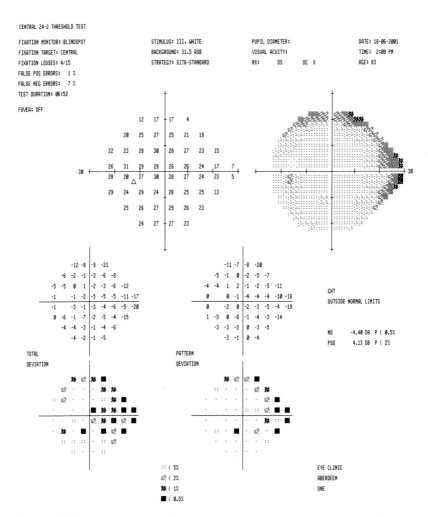

Figure 6.15 The locations with loss of sensitivity are mainly peripheral (see pattern deviation plot), and could not be confirmed in repeated examinations.

With these general guidelines in mind, it is now necessary to apply a systematic approach when facing the visual field printout. The authors' preference includes the following sequence of events:

a) Check the patient's data: refraction (the test should be done using near-vision correction after the age of 40 or after cataract surgery; large refractive errors may induce artifacts), pupil size (ideally greater than 3 mm but, if smaller than 3 mm, at least unchanged from the previous examination), and duration of the test.

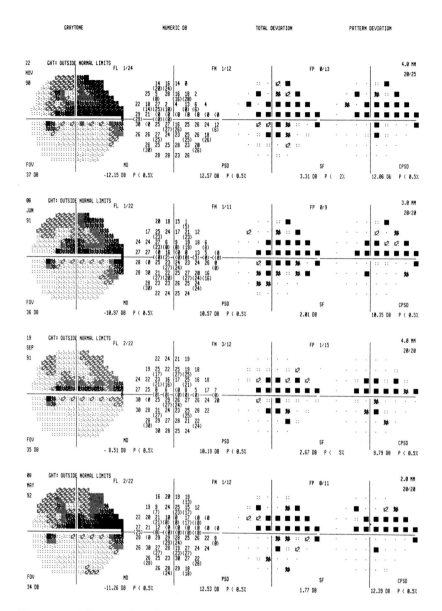

Figure 6.16 Humphrey's printout overview of a patient followed from 1990 to 1992. This is a typical example of long-term fluctuation. Note that there is an apparent improvement in the third visual field, which disappears in the last examination. In fact, the last test is similar to the initial visual field.

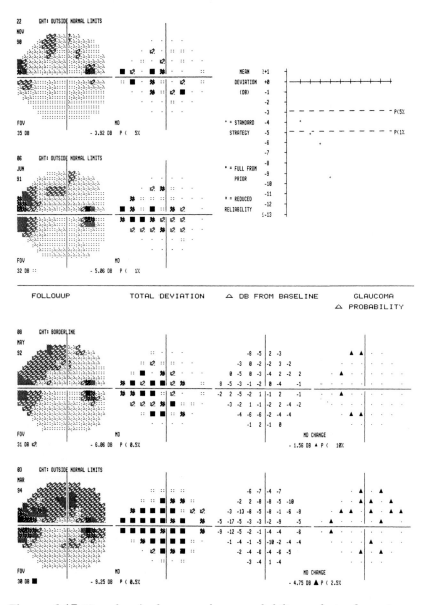

Figure 6.17 Humphrey's glaucoma change probability analysis of a patient followed from 1990 to 1994. The black triangles refer to points where the probability of not having a deterioration is less than 5%. The graph in the right superior area shows a significant reduction in MD (from –3.92 dB in 1990 to –9.25 dB in 1994).

b) Check the reliability indices, observing if the test can be considered reliable.
c) Look at the grayscale, which will allow the visualization of gross defects.
d) Observe the numerical graph to check if suspected areas have low thresholds.
e) Analyse the total deviation probability plot to look for diffuse loss of sensitivity.
f) Look for localized visual field defects (clusters of abnormal points) in the pattern deviation probability plot.
g) Analyse the global indices, particularly the MD (to evaluate the general sensitivity), and the CPSD in full-threshold perimetry, or the PSD if SITA is done (which may confirm the impression of a localized defect).
h) Check the GHT.
i) Compare the visual field to the clinical information.
j) Rule out possible artifacts (e.g. ptosis, edge of the lens rim, inexperienced patient).

The identification of a dense, well-established visual field defect is not a difficult task. The recognition of mild glaucomatous visual field loss, however, requires the establishment of some criteria, among which the following are the most commonly used:

a) Three or more non-edge, adjacent points in the pattern deviation probability plot with $p < 5\%$, one of them with $p < 1\%$.
b) CPSD (or PSD) with $p < 5\%$.
c) GHT outside normal limits.

Other examples of computerized perimetry are shown in Figures 6.18–6.21.

Other forms of perimetry

Short-wavelength automated perimetry (SWAP)

This technique is a modification of automated static threshold perimetry and is available on newer Humphrey models. SWAP uses a yellow background and size V, blue projected stimuli to test the blue cones. The blue cone system is slower and has a low visual acuity (about 20/200). As a consequence, the stimulus is perceived as fuzzy, and the test is more difficult and time-consuming. Uncorrected refractive errors have less of an effect on the thresholds determined by SWAP, but lens opacities tend to result in profoundly depressed fields that are difficult to interpret. SWAP, which comes with statistical analysis software designed to compare the examination with a normative database, has been shown to perform better than standard white-on-white perimetry in the detection of

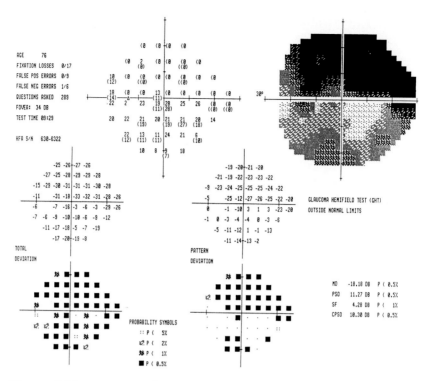

Figure 6.18 Dense, complete superior scotoma in a patient with an inferior notch. Note that fixation is threatened, although the foveal threshold remains normal (34 dB).

early glaucomatous damage. Some reports have also suggested that SWAP may detect progression of a visual field defect earlier than standard automated perimetry. SWAP is indicated in patients with signs or strong risk factors for glaucomatous damage (high IOP, suspicious optic disc, family history), but who have normal white-on-white fields.

Frequency doubling perimetry (FDP)

Based on frequency doubling illusion, this portable instrument presents rapid flickering stimuli to the peripheral visual field. In a normal field, patients perceive twice as many bars as actually exist (Figure 6.22). In abnormal fields, the illusion is present only if the bars are at higher-than-normal contrast levels. The clinical test procedure measures contrast threshold in 19 visual field locations within the central 30 degrees. FDP evaluates the magnocellular pathway (a subset of the retinal ganglion cells) and correlates well with the findings of standard white-on-white perimetry. FDP has been shown to have high

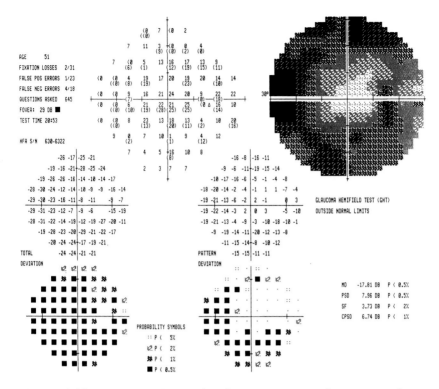

Figure 6.19 Full threshold Humphrey's 30–2 program of a patient with cataract (visual acuity = 20/80) and severe glaucomatous damage. Note that the total deviation probability plot shows more abnormal points than the pattern deviation probability plot, which filters the localized defects caused by glaucoma and discloses both inferior arcuate scotoma and superior nasal step.

sensitivity and specificity for the detection of early glaucomatous damage, and has been proposed as a valid tool for glaucoma screening. It is faster than conventional perimetry (takes about 4 min for full threshold testing), and easier for the patient to perform. However, further studies are necessary to assess the performance of FDP in detecting glaucomatous visual field progression.

High-pass resolution perimetry (HRP)

In high-pass resolution perimetry, rings of different sizes are presented to the peripheral retina. Instead of measuring threshold sensitivity to light, it measures the sensitivity of the retina to the size of the stimulus (i.e., peripheral visual acuity). HRP is believed to detect loss of ganglion cells by finding an increase

91

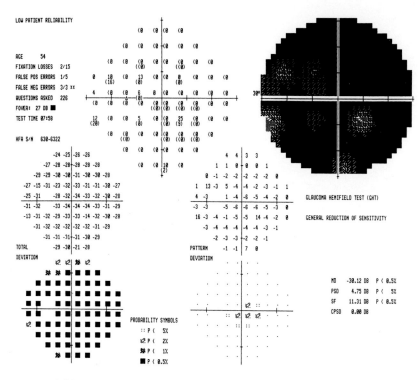

Figure 6.20 Full-threshold Humphrey's 30–2 program of a patient with very severe glaucomatous damage and a transparent lens (visual acuity = 20/80). The gray scale and the total deviation probability plot show a generalized reduction of sensitivity. The numerical grid indicates that almost all points are incapable of seeing the maximum stimulus (< 0 dB). The foveal threshold, however, is 27 dB, indicating that a small central island (of less than 3 degrees of extension) is present. A 10-2 program is better suited to follow this patient's visual field.

in space between these cells. Although the test is rapid, well-accepted by patients, and shows good correlation with standard perimetry, its role in the detection of progression is still unclear.

Other functional tests

Table 6.1 lists other electrophysiological and psychophysical tests that have been used in glaucoma. However, none of the following tests has replaced automated perimetry, which remains the standard psychophysical test for the diagnosis and monitoring of glaucoma patients.

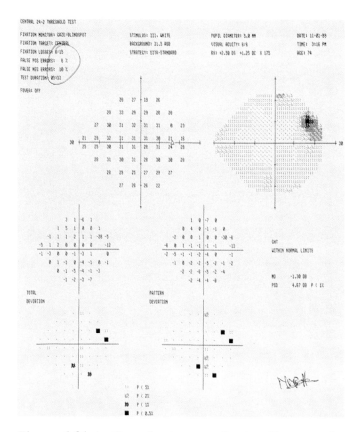

Figure 6.21 Artifact related to poor fixation. Numerous fixation losses (11/15) indicate poor fixation and, therefore, poor reliability of the test. The patient's head was tilted during the test, and the physiological blind spot is represented as a 'scotoma' in the lower temporal region.

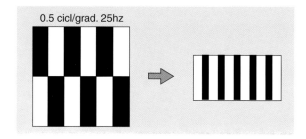

Figure 6.22 In frequency doubling technology (FDT) the test stimulus consists of a sinusoidal spatial waveform composed of alternating white and black stripes (0.25 cycles/degree sinusoidal modulation) than counterphase flicker at 25 Hz. The target is perceived to have twice its actual spatial frequency (frequency-doubling illusion).

Table 6.1 Other functional tests that have been investigated in glaucoma (modified from Choplin NT: *Atlas of glaucoma*, pages 76, 77)

Test	Stimulus	Measurement	Findings in glaucoma
Central contrast sensitivity	Low-contrast flickering stimuli presented to the central 4 degrees	Minimum difference in luminance between stimulus and background of a flickering stimulus	Mean thresholds lower than normal controls
Temporal contrast sensitivity	Stimulus of increasing frequency of flicker presented to the fovea and to the peripheral retina	Intensity of stimulus required to perceive flicker at each presented flicker frequency	Frequency-specific loss at 15 Hz, non-frequency specific mean sensitivity loss greater in glaucoma patients than suspects
Pattern-evoked electro-retinographic response (PERG)	Reversing checkerboard pattern presented on a television screen at varying contrast while standard ERG measurements are obtained	Waveform, latencies of responses and amplitudes of each wave component	Second negative wave selectively depressed in patients with glaucoma
Contrast sensitivity	Figures of decreasing contrast at multiple spatial frequencies	Ability to detect correct orientation of stripe pattern as contrast decreases	Decreased contrast acuity in glaucoma patients, particularly at high spatial frequencies
Motion sensitivity	Patch of dots moving in one direction or motion of a line	Ability to detect movement in the peripheral retina	Decreased ability to detect moving stimuli
Color vision	Farnsworth-Munsell 100 Hue Test, Farnsworth D-15 test, Nagel or Pickford-Nicholson anomaloscope	Defects in color vision	Blue-yellow defects occur early in glaucoma, red-green defects appear with advanced optic neuropathy

Color contrast sensitivity	Computer-driven color television system	Color contrast threshold as the fraction of the maximum color available for color combinations on each color axis	Sensitivity to blue and red lights (relative to green) less than controls
Scotopic retinal sensitivity	Flickering stimulus increasing in luminance in a dark-adapted patient	Sensitivity to flashing light	Reduction in absolute retinal sensitivity
Flicker visual-evoked potential	Flickering stimulus of varying frequencies	Amplitude and phase responses of VEP	Amplitude loss at higher flicker frequencies, correlating with visual field defects
Color pattern-reversal visual-evoked potential	Reversing checkerboard of black-white, black-red, or black-blue	P1-wave peak time and amplitude for each pattern	Decrease in measured parameters compared to normals, especially the black-red and black-blue checkerboards
Visual-evoked potentials (VEP) after photostress	VEP measurements before and after 30 seconds of photostress	Time for VEP recordings to return to baseline	Longer VEP recovery time for glaucoma patients

95

Suggested reading

Anderson DR, Patella M. *Automated static perimetry*, 2nd Edition. St. Louis: CV Mosby, 1992.

Bebie H, Frankhauser F, Spahr J. Static perimetry: accuracy and fluctuations. *Acta Ophthalmol* 1976;**54**:339–48.

Bergtsson B, Heijl A. Inter-subject variability and normal limits of the SITA Standard, SITA Fast, and the Humprey Full Threshold computerized perimetry strategies, SITA STATPAC. *Acta Ophthalmol Scand* 1999;**77**:125–9.

Bergtsson B, Olsson J, Heijl A, Rootzén H. A new generation of algorithms for computerized threshold perimetry, SITA. *Acta Ophthalmol Scand* 1997;**75**:368–75.

Choplin NT. Psychophysical and electrophysiological testing in glaucoma: visual fields and other functional tests. In: Choplin NT, Lundy DC, eds. *Atlas of glaucoma*. London, UK: Martin Dunitz, 1998; 75–102.

Costa VP. *Perimetria Computadorizada*, 2a Edição. Rio de Janeiro, Brasil: Editora Rio Med, 2000.

Flammer J, Drance SM, Augustiny L, Frankhauser A. Quantification of visual field defects with automated perimetry. *Invest Ophthalmol Vis Sci* 1985;**26**:176–80.

Flammer J. The concept of visual field defects. *Graefes Arch Klin Exp Ophthalmol* 1986;**224**:389.

Flammer J. The concept of visual field indices. *Graefes Arch Klin Exp Ophthalmol* 1986;**224**:389–92.

Heijl A. Computer test logics for automatic perimetry. *Acta Ophthalmol* 1977;**155**:837–40.

Heijl A. Humphrey field analyzer. In: Drance SM, Anderson DR (eds). *Automatic perimetry in glaucoma: a practical guide*. Orlando: Grune & Stratton, 1985; 129–48.

Heijl A, Lindgren G, Olsson J. A package for the statistical analysis of computerized fields. In: Greve EL, Heijl A (eds). *Proceedings of the Seventh International Visual Field Symposium*, Amsterdam, September 1986. Hingham: Kluwer Academic Publishers, 1987; 153–64.

Heijl A, Lindgren G, Olsson J. Reliability parameters in computerized perimetry. *Doc Ophthalmol Proc Ser* 1987;**49**:593–7.

Katz J, Sommer A. A longitudinal study of the age-adjusted variability of automated visual fields. *Arch Ophthalmol* 1987;**105**:1083–6.

Katz J, Sommer A, Witt K. Reliability of visual field results over repeated testing. *Ophthalmology* 1991;**98**:70–4.

Keltner JL, Johnson CA. Screening for visual field abnormalities with automated perimetry. *Surv Ophthalmol* 1983;**28**:175–80.

Mikelberg FS, Drance SM. The mode of progression of visual field defects in glaucoma. *Am J Ophthalmol* 1984;**98**:443–7.

Schmidt T, Fischer FW: The Goldmann perimeter: forty years of development. *Klin Mbl Augenheilk* 1988;**193**:237–45.

Sommer A, Enger C, Witt K. Screening for glaucomatous visual field loss with automated threshold perimetry. *Am J Ophthalmol* 1987;**103**:681–5.

Tate GW Jr. The physiological basis for perimetry. In: Drance SM, Anderson DR (eds). *Automated perimetry in glaucoma. A practical guide.* Orlando: Grune & Stratton Inc., 1985; 1–28.

Werner EB. *Manual of visual fields.* New York: Churchill Livingstone Inc., 1991.

SECTION II
CLINICAL ENTITIES

7. CHRONIC OR PRIMARY OPEN ANGLE GLAUCOMA

Augusto Azuara-Blanco, Richard P Wilson, and Vital P Costa

Introduction

In the ophthalmology literature and in clinical practice, idiopathic open-angle glaucomas tend to be classified into chronic or primary open-angle glaucoma (POAG) and normal-tension glaucoma (NTG) or low-tension glaucoma (LTG). These two subtypes are defined on the basis of intraocular pressure. For example, a patient with open-angle glaucoma and with an untreated intraocular pressure below 21 mmHg (confirmed with multiple IOP measurements at different times of the day) is considered to have NTG. However, it is not clear whether the use of this arbitrarily selected parameter has somehow successfully identified two different disease entities.

Chronic or primary open-angle glaucoma (POAG) is the most common form of glaucoma and is characterized by the following four findings: (1) an intraocular pressure (IOP) above 21 mmHg; (2) an open, normal appearing anterior chamber angle; (3) no ocular or systemic abnormality that might account for the raised IOP; and (4) typical glaucomatous visual field and/or optic nerve damage. This type of glaucoma is likely to represent a spectrum of disorders in which several causative factors have varying degrees of influence.

Epidemiology

Glaucoma is the leading cause of irreversible blindness throughout the world. It has been estimated that during this decade glaucoma will be the second largest cause of bilateral blindness in the world (6.7 million people), only surpassed by cataract.

In the USA, about 2.5 million people have glaucoma, and 130 000 people are blind because of this disease. Since most people with glaucoma do not become functionally blind, the significant visual loss before blindness and its potential effect on functional status is not accounted for by current statistics on blindness.

Chronic or primary open-angle glaucoma accounts for most cases of glaucoma, although in some ethnic groups chronic angle closure glaucoma (ACG) can be the most common form of the disease. In whites, open-angle glaucoma is uncommon in young individuals. In white adults (older than 40 years), population-based studies in several European countries and in the USA have consistently reported a prevalence of glaucoma between 1.1% and 2.1%. The prevalence of glaucoma increases with age (see below). In those of African origin, the prevalence of pOAG is three or four times higher than in whites, and the disease tends to behave more aggressively and manifest at an earlier age. Glaucoma is the leading cause of blindness among African-Americans.

Since there are heterogeneous groups of people in Asia, population-based prevalence data on glaucoma is limited and difficult to interpret. In the Chinese, angle closure glaucoma is the predominant type, outnumbering all other types combined. However, a population-based survey in Japan reported a prevalence of pOAG of 2.62%, and only 0.34% of ACG. Interestingly, most Japanese patients with pOAG have normal-tension glaucoma.

Risk factors

Identification of risk factors has preventive and therapeutic implications in glaucoma. Some risk factors (e.g. IOP) may be causative and changeable, and strategies to modify these risk factors can help to prevent the disease. Other risk factors (age, race, family history) are not changeable but are useful for identifying individuals for whom medical examination is advisable or medical treatment is indicated. The known risk factors for glaucoma are:

1   Intraocular pressure. This is the main risk factor for the development of glaucoma. 10% of those with raised IOP have visual field loss and 15–40% of ocular hypertensives develop field loss within 10 years. In general, the higher the IOP, the greater the likelihood of glaucoma. A causal role for IOP is supported by experimental studies and clinical and epidemiological observations. However, many eyes with IOP above the average range do not develop glaucoma. Conversely, many eyes with IOP within the normal range develop glaucoma.
2   Age. The older a person is, the greater the chance of having glaucoma. Prevalence estimates have generally been three to eight times higher in the oldest age groups than in the 40–50 year age group.
3   Race. There is a higher prevalence of glaucoma in those of African descent than in whites (three or four times higher).
4   Family history. Individuals who have a first-degree relative (parent, sibling, or offspring) with glaucoma have greater risk (at least 10–30%) of developing the disease.
5   Myopia and diabetes appear to be risk factors for glaucoma, although the supporting evidence is not strong.

6 Some studies have suggested systemic hypertension, migraine and vasospasm as risk factors for some types of glaucoma. However, further data are needed to confirm this association.

Clinical features and diagnosis

In most cases, POAG develops in middle life or later. Because of the insidious and painless nature of POAG, patients often do not report symptoms unless there is severe optic nerve damage and visual loss. The cornea is clear, the anterior chamber is deep and, by definition, the anterior chamber angle looks open and normal. Although outflow facility is reduced in POAG, tonography is no longer an integral part of the standard clinical assessment.

The IOP is typically raised. However, the diagnosis of POAG cannot be made on the basis of IOP, which is associated with low sensitivity (70%) and specificity (30%). A mean IOP of 16 ± 2.5 mmHg (range 10–21 mmHg) is seen in the general population. The interval between 11 and 21 mmHg was thought to include 95% of the population, and an IOP measuring 21 mmHg was formerly considered to be the cutoff between normality and glaucoma. However, the IOP distribution in the general population is not Gaussian, being skewed to the right (i.e. there are more people with pressures in the low twenties than would have been predicted by Gaussian statistics). The chance of discovering glaucomatous damage on examination of the optic disc or visual field increases with IOP across the entire range.

Assessment of the optic nerve and retinal nerve fiber layer (RNFL) is critical in determining the presence of POAG. Changes in the optic nerve (Figure 7.1) and RNFL will often precede any changes in perimetry. The clinical characteristics of glaucomatous optic neuropathy are described in Chapter 5. When changes in the optic disc are assessed, non-glaucomatous entities such

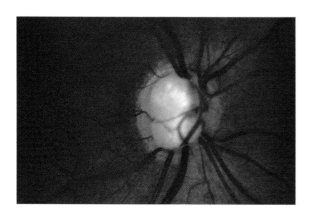

Figure 7.1
Advanced generalized cupping as a result of primary open angle glaucoma.

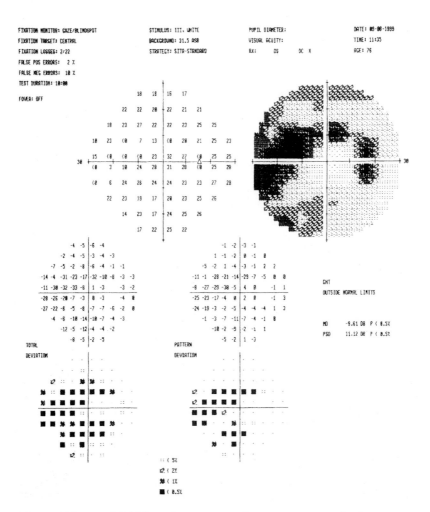

Figure 7.2 Visual field loss characteristic of primary open angle glaucoma. There is a superior arcuate scotoma, associated with a superior nasal step.

as ischemic optic neuropathy, compressive lesions, and congenital anomalies such as optic pits and tilted discs must be included in the differential diagnosis. Additional ocular signs may be useful in the diagnosis of POAG. An afferent pupillary defect can be observed if the glaucomatous damage is asymmetrical.

Visual field loss is the third sign of glaucoma (Figure 7.2). For the diagnosis of glaucoma, one usually requires two of the three signs, e.g. raised IOP and disc changes, or disc and visual field changes in the absence of raised IOP.

Typically, POAG is a bilateral disease. Asymmetry of IOP and optic nerve damage is common, although advanced abnormalities in one eye with an entirely normal fellow eye suggest a different diagnosis (ocular trauma, steroid-induced glaucoma, exfoliation syndrome, ICE syndrome, inflammatory glaucoma, etc.).

Normal-tension glaucoma

Normal-tension glaucoma is not uncommon, and it may account for up to 20–30% of all non-Asian patients with chronic open-angle glaucoma. In Japan, chronic open-angle glaucoma is most commonly associated with low IOP (i.e. NTG).

Is NTG fundamentally different from POAG? The Normal Tension Glaucoma Study Group reported that reduction of 30% from baseline IOP is effective in slowing the progression of NTG, suggesting a role for IOP in the pathogenesis of NTG. However, many untreated patients (40%) did not show progression of damage after 5 years of follow-up, whereas 20% of the treated group showed progression despite a 30% reduction in IOP.

Blood flow has been judged important in the pathogenesis of NTG. Patients with NTG tend to show a higher incidence of vasoespastic manifestations such as migraine and Raynaud's. Multiple studies have assessed the ocular and systemic circulations, although all methods used to measure ocular blood flow have limitations. Most of them suggest that the ocular circulation may be compromised in patients with NTG, but it is not clear whether these changes are pathogenetically important or if they are epiphenomena.

It seems that eyes with NTG have different structural characteristics of the optic nerve than eyes with POAG. The optic disc rim tends to be thinner in NTG, and the cupping and disc area are larger (Figure 7.3). In NTG there is an increased prevalence of acquired pits of the optic nerve and disc hemorrhages

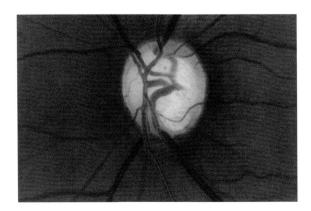

Figure 7.3 Large optic disc with moderately advanced cupping, with preferential loss of inferior and nasal rim.

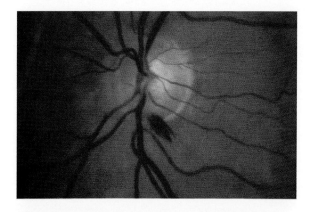

Figure 7.4 Flame-shaped disc hemorrhage. Characteristic appearance and location of a flame-shaped hemorrhage in the infero-temporal portion of the optic disc.

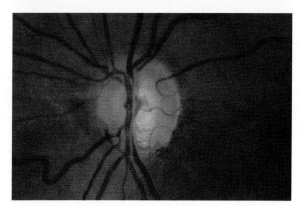

Figure 7.5 Localized inferior notch of the optic disc in a patient with normal tension glaucoma.

(Figure 7.4). NTG may be associated with more focal loss than POAG (Figure 7.5), and deep scotomas close to fixation may be more common in NTG than in POAG (Figure 7.6). Eyes with NTG have been shown to have significantly thinner corneas than eyes with POAG. Because applanation tonometry of a thinner cornea results in an inaccurately low measured IOP, it is possible that some cases of NTG may be misclassified.

Several immune-related serum abnormalities are more common among patients with NTG than in those with POAG. This suggests that immune factors may play a part in the pathogenesis of some cases of NTG.

We think that the typical damage of NTG may have several different causes, but we are not able to characterize and differentiate them. The view of POAG and NTG as single entities is no longer valid. In light of contemporary knowledge, it does not appear appropriate to dichotomize glaucoma on the basis of IOP alone. It appears more accurate to consider glaucoma as a disorder with characteristic optic nerve damage resulting in characteristic visual field loss in which IOP is variably a risk factor. The identification of the different

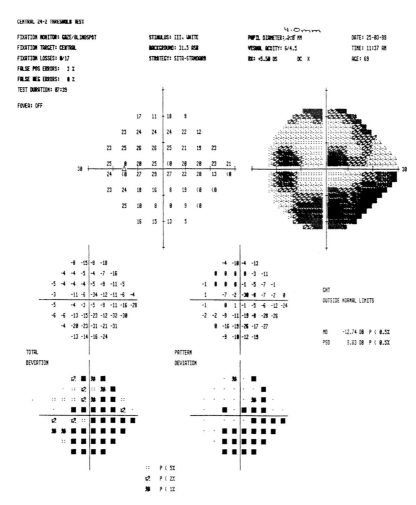

Figure 7.6 Superior dense paracentral scotoma in a patient with normal-tension glaucoma.

pathophysiological mechanisms of damage is mandatory to truly understand POAG and NTG.

From the practical point of view, we could apply the information provided by the Normal Tension-Glaucoma Study as follows: it is quite helpful to determine whether the disease is progressive and, if so, the rate of progression. In progressive cases, treatment should be initiated. However, if there is already severe damage, observation to detect progression would not be advisable. In these cases, lowering the IOP is attempted as the benefits of treatment outweighs its risks. Medical therapy and laser treatment can be effective in minimizing progression of the disease. In many cases, however, filtration surgery will be

8. Primary Angle Closure Glaucoma

Augusto Azuara-Blanco, Richard P Wilson, and Vital P Costa

Angle closure glaucomas: introduction

Angle closure glaucomas are characterized by temporary or permanent contact of peripheral iris against the trabecular meshwork, resulting in obstruction of aqueous outflow. The clinical presentation can be acute (Figure 8.1) or chronic.

The most common mechanism of angle closure glaucoma is *pupillary block* (e.g. primary angle closure glaucoma and secondary pupillary block glaucomas). Under normal conditions, contact between the iris and the lens results in a relative obstruction to the flow of aqueous from the posterior to the anterior chamber, causing a higher pressure of aqueous in the posterior chamber, and pushing the iris forward (Figure 8.2). This phenomenon is called *relative pupillary block*. An increased pupillary block and increased pressure of the posterior chamber causes a forward displacement of the peripheral iris that may close the anterior chamber angle and raise the IOP, originating angle closure glaucoma (See Chapter 4).

Angle closure glaucoma can be induced by other mechanisms that lead to an anterior displacement of the iris (e.g. plateau iris syndrome, aqueous misdirection, scleral buckling surgery, tumors, cysts), or by tissues or membranes that obstruct the outflow pathway directly (e.g. neovascular glaucoma, ICE syndrome, inflammatory debris; see Chapter 9).

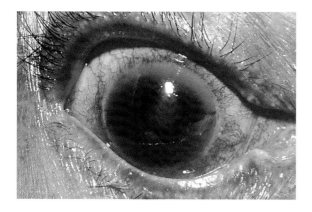

Figure 8.1 Acute angle closure glaucoma. This patient with acute phakic pupillary block presented with blurred vision, pain and redness. The intraocular pressure was 64 mmHg.

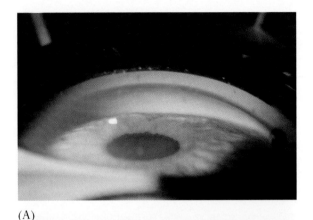

(A)

Figure 8.2 In pupillary block, peripheral iris is placed anteriorly because of the force of the aqueous behind it (A). During indentation, the peripheral iris can move posteriorly with the force of indentation (B).

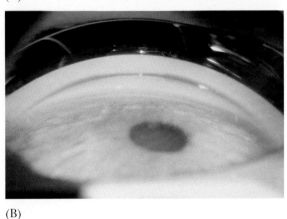

(B)

Epidemiology

The prevalence and presentation of primary angle closure glaucoma greatly varies in different ethnic groups. The prevalence over age 40 years is 0.1% in whites, less than 0.1% in blacks, 1.4% in Chinese, and 2.65% in Inuit Eskimos. Blacks, Asians and Eskimos frequently present free of symptoms with chronic angle closure glaucoma.

In Asians, chronic angle closure glaucoma may be more prevalent than open-angle glaucoma.

Primary angle closure glaucoma

Acute primary angle closure glaucoma

Hyperopic eyes with small anterior segments are predisposed to pupillary block and attacks of angle closure. This is more common in women because of their shallower anterior chamber, especially after 50 years of age. Increased relative pupillary block due to thickening and anterior displacement of the lens associated with ageing may further compromise an already narrow angle. A mid-dilated pupil caused by dim light, stress, and use of anticholinergic or sympathomimetic agents may result in pupillary block and precipitate an angle closure attack.

Diagnosis

Patients present with a sudden, usually unilateral onset of severe ocular pain, decreased vision, halos around lights, and redness (Figure 8.1). The acute rise in IOP (often more than 50 mmHg) may produce autonomic stimulation and induce nausea, vomiting, bradychardia, and sweating.

The cornea shows epithelial edema and, sometimes, stromal thickening and folds in Descemet's membrane. The anterior chamber is shallow, especially peripherally. Moderate anterior chamber inflammation is common, and the pupil appears mid-dilated and nonreactive or sluggish. Occasionally, sector atrophy of the iris may appear from pressure-related ischemia. The lens may show anterior subcapsular opacities, called Glaukomflecken.

Adequate visualization of the angle by gonioscopy may not be possible because of corneal edema, although topical glycerin and a reduction in IOP may help to clear the cornea. When the view is adequate, the anterior chamber angle appears to be closed. It may be possible to open the angle with indentation gonioscopy and document the presence and extent of peripheral anterior synechiae.

The optic disc may appear normal or hyperemic during the attack. Several months after an attack, pallor of the optic disc without cupping typically appears.

Examination of the fellow eye is important to the diagnosis of angle-closure glaucoma as usually it also is narrow (Figure 4.2, Chapter 4). This is especially important if corneal edema prevents an adequate view of the eye having the attack.

Treatment

An acute attack constitutes a medical emergency. The first goal is to break the attack, usually with medical therapy. Attempts should then be made to relieve the pupillary block with laser iridotomy, and to treat the fellow eye.

Initial medical therapy includes the administration of oral or intravenous acetazolamide (500 mg), topical aqueous suppressants (betablocker, carbonic anhydrase inhibitor, alpha-2 agonist), and topical pilocarpine (1–2%, twice over 30 min). Frequent topical corticosteroids are also started. If the attack is not broken, an osmotic agent is given (oral 50% glycerin, oral 45% isosorbide, or intravenous 20% mannitol, 1–2g/kg).

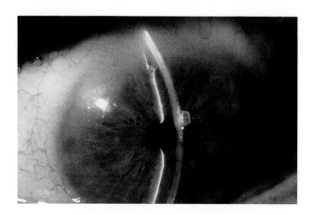

Figure 8.3 Laser peripheral iridotomy, clinical photograph. The anterior chamber is shallow, and the peripheral iridotomy is located at 11 o'clock.

In recalcitrant cases, Nd:YAG iridotomy (Figure 8.3), argon laser irido-plasty, or corneal compression can be tried to break the acute attack (see Chapter 12).

Permanent relief of pupillary block is achieved with *Nd:YAG laser peripheral iridotomy* (see Chapter 12), which is most easily done after the attack has resolved. If laser iridotomy is not possible, argon laser gonioplasty or surgical peripheral iridectomy is indicated.

After an attack, the anterior chamber angle may appear open or may show peripheral anterior synechiae to a variable extent. If the amount of angle closure precludes the maintenance of a normal intraocular pressure with medication, *surgical goniosynechialysis* can be used to mechanically open the angle. It is usually done with a broad and blunt iris spatula, and may open the angle if accomplished within 6–12 months of the onset of angle closure.

The term '*combined mechanism glaucoma*' refers to eyes where there appears to be both an angle closure and open angle mechanism to the glaucoma. Examples include eyes of patients with an open angle and uncontrolled IOP after an acute angle closure glaucoma attack has been broken, and those in which peripheral anterior synechia are present but not enough to explain the degree of raised IOP. Medical therapy and filtering surgery may be needed to control the IOP.

The fellow eye should undergo prompt prophylactic laser iridotomy to prevent an acute attack.

Prevention

Nd:YAG peripheral iridotomy should be considered to treat patients with narrow anterior chamber angles that appear to be occludable or with appositional angle closure on gonioscopy. In patients with possibly occludable angles and a history

114

of symptoms or signs of previous episodes of acute or subacute angle closure, laser iridotomy is recommended. To decide whether laser iridotomy is required, some clinicians use provocative tests in which patients adopt a prone position, with stimulation of mydriasis and/or a dark room. A test is considered positive when the IOP rises by 8 mmHg or more. However, the positive and negative predictive values of such tests are not high enough to recommend their routine application.

Subacute and chronic primary angle closure glaucoma

Some patients describe transitory episodes of ocular discomfort, blurred vision or colored halos around lights which, in the presence of a narrow angle, are suggestive of *subacute angle closure glaucoma*. These symptoms typically occur at night and dissappear spontaneously by the following morning, probably due to the miosis of sleep. Repeated subacute attacks may result in the development of permanent peripheral anterior synechiae and chronic angle closure glaucoma. The synechiae tend to be broad based, and are most commonly seen in the superior quadrant.

Creeping angle closure glaucoma is another form of chronic angle closure glaucoma, in which the anterior chamber angle narrows progressively over time. This form of glaucoma is the most common form of angle closure glaucoma in black patients, especially in those on miotic therapy.

Diagnosis

Patients with chronic angle closure glaucoma may be symptom-free or may refer to symptoms compatible with subacute angle closure. The diagnosis is based on gonioscopy (Figure 8.4). Indentation gonioscopy is vital to differentiate parts of the angle with appositional or permanent closure.

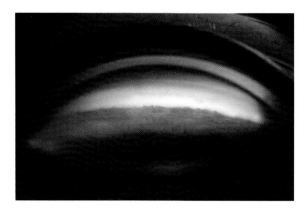

Figure 8.4 Chronic angle closure glaucoma. Despite indentation gonioscopy, iridotrabecular apposition persists, indicating synechial closure.

Treatment

Laser peripheral iridotomy should be done in all cases. If more than one quadrant of the anterior chamber angle has appositional closure and opens with indentation gonioscopy, laser iridotomy may cure the disease.

The level of IOP and the need for further medical treatment depend on the extension of peripheral anterior synechiae and the function of the remaining anterior chamber angle. Medical treatment and filtering surgery in patients with angle closure glaucoma are addressed in the relevant chapters.

Other pupillary block glaucomas

Conditions that may lead to secondary pupillary block include a subluxated or dislocated lens, an anterior chamber intraocular lens in an eye with no patent peripheral iridectomy, iris contact with the anterior vitreous face, and a secluded pupil with 360 degrees of posterior synechiae from previous inflammation. There is often a prominent iris bombee, with the iris coming into direct apposition with the peripheral cornea.

Treatment

Medical treatment is undertaken only as a temporizing measure. By vigorous dilation and the use of aqueous suppressants the pupillary block may be broken and the IOP lowered. The most effective treatment is a Nd:YAG laser iridectomy or, if not possible, surgical peripheral iridectomy or trabeculectomy. At the same time, the underlying cause should be addressed (e.g. inflammation, vitreous in the anterior chamber).

Plateau iris

'Plateau iris *configuration*' refers to the presence of a flat iris configuration with an abrupt posterior turn near the iris insertion. This leads to a narrow angle in the presence of an unusually deep central anterior chamber. Most eyes with plateau iris configuration show a relative pupillary block. Hence, laser iridotomy may ameliorate the plateau iris configuration and widen the anterior chamber angle. If laser iridotomy does not affect the positioning and shape of the iris and the anterior chamber angle, the term used to describe this condition is 'plateau iris *syndrome*'. This syndrome is related to an abnormal anterior position and size of the ciliary processes, which push the iris forward (Figure 8.5). Patients with plateau iris may develop acute or chronic angle closure.

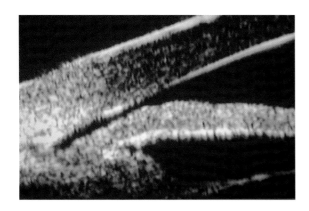

Figure 8.5 Plateau iris syndrome, ultrasound biomicroscopy. In plateau iris syndrome, the anteriorly placed ciliary body forces the peripheral iris into the angle. The iris contour is planar centrally, and the angle is barely open.

Diagnosis

Plateau iris is suspected initially based on gonioscopy and slit-lamp examination. Unlike primary angle closure due to pupillary block, the central anterior chamber depth is not shallow.

Treatment

Patients with plateau iris configuration should undergo laser peripheral iridotomy. If gonioscopy still reveals a plateau iris configuration or the anterior chamber angle does not deepen after laser treatment, chronic miotic therapy or laser peripheral iridoplasty or 'gonioplasty' (see Chapter 12) are indicated to prevent angle closure.

Suggested reading

Azuara-Blanco A, Spaeth GL, Araujo SV et al. Plateau iris syndrome associated with multiple ciliary body cysts. *Arch Ophthalmol* 1996;**114**:666.

Forbes M. Indentation gonioscopy and efficacy of iridectomy in angle-closure glaucoma. *Trans Am Ophthalmol Soc* 1974;**74**:488–515.

Pavlin CJ, Ritch R, Foster FS. Ultrasound biomicroscopy in plateau iris syndrome. *Am J Ophthalmol* 1992;**113**:390.

Rith R. Argon laser treatment for medically unresponsive attacks of angle-closure glaucoma. *Am J Ophthalmol* 1982;**94**:197.

Shingleton BJ, Chang MA, Bellows AR et al. Surgical goniosynechiolysis for angle-closure glaucoma. *Ophthalmology* 1990;**97**:551.

Wand M, Grant WM, Simmons RJ et al. Plateau iris syndrome. *Trans Am Acad Ophthalmol Otolaryngol* 1977;**83**:122–30.

Wand M. Argon laser gonioplasty for synechial angle closure. *Arch Ophthalmol* 1992;**110**:363–7.

Weiss HS, Shingleton BJ, Goode SM et al. Argon laser gonioplasty in the treatment of angle-closure glaucoma. *Am J Ophthalmol* 1992;**114**:14.

9. SECONDARY GLAUCOMAS
Vital P Costa, Richard P Wilson, and Augusto Azuara-Blanco

Definition

Secondary glaucoma applies to cases in which the intraocular pressure (IOP) is raised through mechanisms other than primary dysfunction of the trabecular meshwork. The mechanisms that raise IOP are used to define secondary glaucoma.

Exfoliation syndrome

Exfoliation syndrome is characterized by the deposition of grayish-white material on the anterior lens capsule, pupil margin, iris, corneal endothelium, zonular fibers, ciliary body, and the trabecular meshwork. This disorder, however, is not limited to the eye, since the same material has been found in the conjunctiva, orbital blood vessels, lung, liver, kidney, skin, and cerebral meninges. Histology has shown that the flaky material is made of glycosaminoglycans, synthesized by an abnormal basement membrane. The disease should be differentiated from capsular delamination, characterized by true exfoliation of the lens capsule and typically seen in glassblowers whose eyes are exposed to high temperatures. Raised IOP, which is seen in about 22–50% of cases, is thought to occur secondarily to the accumulation of pigment and exfoliation material in the trabecular meshwork, reducing conventional outflow.

Exfoliation syndrome is a common cause of secondary open-angle glaucoma in many populations, although it may be associated with narrow angles in 30% of cases. It causes about 50% of glaucoma cases in Iceland and Finland, and 10% of glaucoma in the USA. Exfoliation glaucoma is typically bilateral, although often asymmetrical, and is usually more aggressive, with higher IOPs than primary open angle glaucoma (POAG). The incidence of exfoliation typically increases with age, and is more common in the sixth and seventh decades, especially among women.

The anterior capsule of the lens presents with three distinct zones: a central, translucent disc with curled edges surrounded by a clear zone, and a peripheral granular zone (Figure 9.1). The movement of the iris with pupillary excursions across the rough exfoliation material on the anterior lens capsule results in pigment dispersion from the iris pigment epithelium and increased flare from

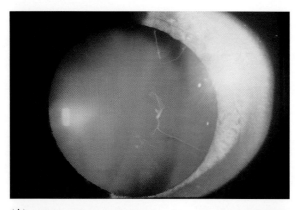

Figure 9.1A and 9.1B Deposition of exfoliation material on the anterior lens capsule.

(A)

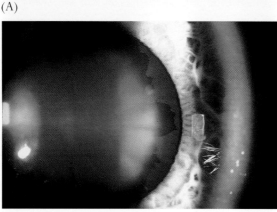

(B)

the abraided posterior surface of the iris. Transillumination defects are usually seen in the pupillary margin, and deposition of pigment is observed throughout the anterior segment, including the trabecular meshwork. Pigment may also be deposited on or sometimes anterior to Schwalbe's line, creating a wavy line (Sampaolesi's line). The presence of pigment deposition in the superior angle, associated with loss of the pupillary ruff in an elderly patient, is highly suggestive of exfoliation syndrome.

Even though the approach to medical treatment in exfoliation glaucoma is similar to that of POAG, it fails earlier and more frequently than the latter. Argon laser trabeculoplasty is a successful treatment option, but may be associated with a higher incidence of postoperative IOP spikes. The attachment of zonular fibers to the lens may be weakened in patients with exfoliation syndrome, making cataract surgery more difficult and increasing the chances of vitreous loss. Trabeculectomy is associated with success rates similar to those obtained in POAG.

Pigmentary glaucoma

Pigmentary glaucoma is a secondary open-angle glaucoma associated with the pigment dispersion syndrome (PDS). Although most cases of pigment dispersion syndrome are sporadic, an autosomal dominant pattern has been described and a locus identified in chromosome 7. The disorder is characterized by chafing of the peripheral iris against the anterior lens zonules, to cause the release of pigment from the posterior pigment epithelium. Current thinking on the pathophysiology involves the presence of a reverse pupillary block. With susceptible individuals, each blink compresses the cornea, sending a wave of fluid across the anterior chamber and knocking the lens posteriorly against the elastic tether of the zonules. The anterior chamber volume is increased, causing a momentary relatively lower pressure in this chamber compared with the posterior chamber. Aqueous is drawn into the anterior chamber until the lens is pulled back against the pupil, trapping an abnormally increased volume of aqueous in the anterior chamber. The peripheral iris is pushed back against the zonules, resulting in zonular–iris chafe and pigment dispersion.

PDS typically occurs in young, white, male patients with myopia. Asian and black patients are rarely affected by this disorder, possibly because their irides are thicker and less flaccid. PDS tends to decrease with age, since the lens axial diameter increases and keeps the peripheral iris away from the zonular fibers.

Once the pigment is released, it may accumulate in other areas of the anterior segment, including:

a) Corneal endothelium – the pigment is phagocytized by the endothelial cells, forming a vertical spindle that can be seen at the slit lamp (Krukenberg spindle).
b) Trabecular meshwork – the pigment is carried by the aqueous humor and accumulates in the trabecular meshwork, creating a heavily pigmented band that extends for 360 degrees (Figure 9.2). Pigment may also be deposited anterior to Schwalbe's line.

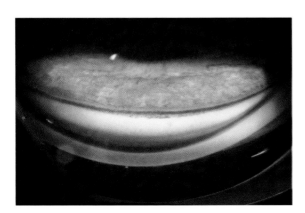

Figure 9.2
Gonioscopy of a patient with pigmentary glaucoma. Observe the dense, dark band at the trabecular meshwork level.

121

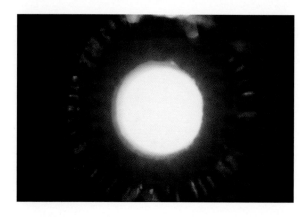

Figure 9.3 Iris transillumination defects in a patient with pigmentary dispersion syndrome.

c) Iris stroma.
d) Posterior lens surface – the pigment may create a ring at Weigert's ligament, which can be seen when the pupil is dilated.

The continuous release of pigment generates transillumination defects in the peripheral iris that tend to coalesce as the dispersion increases (Figure 9.3). Although glaucoma is thought to be secondary to the accumulation of pigment in the trabecular meshwork, it is unclear why all patients with PDS do not end up developing pigmentary glaucoma. About one third of patients with PDS will develop pigmentary glaucoma over 15 years. Patients with pigmentary glaucoma typically show IOP spikes after exercise and pupil dilatation.

All antiglaucoma drugs can be used to treat pigmentary glaucoma, although miotics have the advantage of contracting the iris and bridging the posterior surface up and away from the zonular fibers, reducing pigment dispersion. However, even with longer-release preparations, miotics are not well tolerated by young myopic patients. Furthermore, these patients are also at increased risk for retinal detachment when treated with miotics. Although latanoprost may result in iris pigmentation, it does not exacerbate pigment dispersion, since this side-effect is caused by an increased concentration of melanin in the iris stroma, not affecting the iris epithelium.

Although argon laser trabeculoplasty is highly effective in the short term, more than 50% of patients show failure after 5 years. Laser iridotomy has been suggested as a prophylactic treatment, since it relieves reverse pupillary block and inhibits the development of posterior iris concavity. However, it does not completely eliminate exercise-induced pigment dispersion, and there are no long-term studies to show that it effectively reduces pigment dispersion and improves IOP control.

Guarded filtration procedures can be done in patients who do not respond to medical or laser treatment. Although most patients are young, antimetabolites should be used with caution, since myopic patients are at a greater risk of developing hypotony maculopathy.

Corticosteroid-induced glaucoma

The use of any corticosteroid (topical, inhalational, systemic, periocular, or endogenous) may result in raised IOP and development of a secondary open-angle glaucoma. IOP increase occurs between 2 and 6 weeks after the initiation of steroids, and depends on the potency, duration, and type of treatment (topical steroids are more likely to cause glaucoma than systemic steroids). Patients with POAG are more likely to show steroid-induced IOP increase (45–90%) than the general population (5–10% by 6 weeks). After 6 months of topical dexamethasone usage, however, more than 50% of the latter will show some IOP increase.

The mechanisms that reduce conventional outflow involved in steroid-induced glaucoma include:

a) The accumulation of glycosaminoglycans in the juxtacanalicular space.
b) Decreased capacity for phagocytosis by the endothelial cells in the trabecular meshwork, mediated by membrane stabilization.

The diagnosis is confirmed when the corticosteroid is discontinued and the IOP decreases. Alternatively, challenging the fellow eye (in unilateral cases) with topical steroids may be attempted. Typically, the IOP tends to fall back to normal values 2–4 weeks after interruption of steroids, but some cases with long-term steroid therapy may persist with high IOPs long after the discontinuation.

Medical therapy is used to treat steroid-induced glaucoma. Steroids are discontinued or, if not possible, reduced. Occasionally, it may be necessary to excise a depot of periocular steroid if this has caused severe raised IOP. Argon laser trabeculoplasty can be done, although success rates are generally lower than in POAG, exfoliation glaucoma and pigmentary glaucoma. Filtration surgery may be indicated in refractory cases.

Traumatic glaucoma

Penetrating and non-penetrating injuries of the eye may both lead to glaucoma. Blunt trauma frequently causes equatorial stretching and intraocular lesions that affect the seven ocular rings (as suggested by Campbell):

a) Pupil sphincter tears.

123

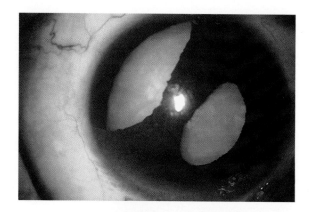

Figure 9.4
Iridodialysis and cataract in a patient with glaucoma secondary to trauma.

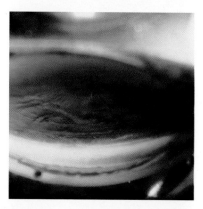

Figure 9.5
Traumatic angle recession. Observe the asymmetry between the right side of the picture (normal angle) and the left side, where the angle recession is visualized.

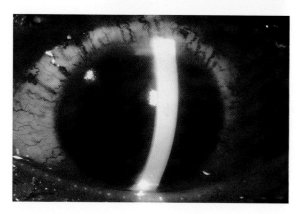

Figure 9.6
Traumatic hyphema occupying 7/8 of the anterior chamber.

b) Iridodialysis, a complete separation of the iris from the ciliary body (Figure 9.4).

c) Cyclodialysis, resulting in a cleft located between the ciliary body and the sclera.

d) Angle recession, characterized by a tear in the face of the ciliary body, frequently between the longitudinal and circular muscles of the ciliary body (Figure 9.5).
e) Trabecular dialysis, creating a flap in the trabecular meshwork.
f) Disruption of the zonules, leading to lens luxation or subluxation.
g) Retinal dialysis, which may be followed by a retinal detachment.

Blunt traumas may also cause rupture of the major arterial circle of the iris, resulting in hyphemas. The amount of blood may vary from a microhyphema (visualized by gonioscopy) to a total hyphema occupying the entire anterior chamber (Figure 9.6). After the injury, IOP may be increased by several mechanisms, including mechanical obstruction of the trabecular meshwork by red blood cells, anterior chamber inflammation, direct trauma to the meshwork, trauma to the lens with rupture of the capsule, and pupillary block (by vitreous or by a dislocated lens). On the other hand, IOP may also be reduced following trauma, either by decreased aqueous production (sometimes observed with anterior chamber inflammation), or by increased uveoscleral outflow caused by a cyclodialysis cleft or inflammation.

Patients with hyphema are at risk of three complications: rebleed, secondary glaucoma, and corneal staining. Rebleed usually occurs between the 3rd and 5th day after trauma, and is associated with more severe hyphemas and raised IOP. The risk for early IOP increase is proportional to the amount of blood and to the extension of the angle recession, which commonly accompanies a hyphema. Aminocaproic acid reduces the rate of rebleeding and should be considered in high-risk eyes. Corneal staining may lead to reduced visual acuity and generally clears over months, starting at the periphery. Evacuation of a hyphema is indicated when the IOP is excessively high and does not respond to medical therapy, or when there are signs of corneal staining (especially in children who can develop amblyopia). Patients with sickle-cell hemoglobinopathy require aggressive management, since the optic nerve is more susceptible to marginal IOP increase. Additionally, acetazolamide should be avoided since it causes metabolic acidosis and stimulates falcization.

Traumatic glaucoma may also develop years after the injury. In this case, it is suggested that traumatic changes in the anterior chamber angle may not be enough to cause IOP increase immediately after the injury. However, when age-related changes in the trabecular meshwork develop in addition to the previous damage, outflow facility may decrease and IOP may increase. The incidence of glaucoma appears to be related to the extent of the angle recession, especially if more than two quadrants are affected. Nevertheless, the angle recession does not directly cause the glaucoma. It is only indicative of the possible microstructural changes induced by the trauma to the trabecular meshwork. It should be noted that miotics and laser trabeculoplasty are not effective treatments.

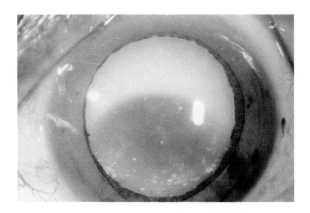

Figure 9.7
Phacolytic glaucoma
in a patient with a
Morganian cataract.
Observe the whitish
precipitates in the
anterior lens capsule.

Lens-induced glaucoma

Phacolytic glaucoma

This secondary open-angle glaucoma develops in the presence of a mature or hypermature cataract (Figure 9.7). In this situation, high-molecular-weight proteins leak into the aqueous humor through microscopic defects in the anterior or posterior lens capsule, and cause a severe obstruction to aqueous outlflow. Although macrophages are seen in the anterior chamber in response to the presence of lens material, they do not seem to cause increased IOP.

Patients with phacolytic glaucoma present with acutely raised IOP, conjunctival and episcleral injection, and pain. On slit-lamp examination, the cornea may be edematous, and the anterior chamber shows an intense flare, occasionally accompanied by a hypopyon. Large white hyperrefringent particles are seen in the anterior chamber. On gonioscopy, the angle is open, although 25% of cases may show concomitant angle-recession. The condition is typically unilateral and affects eyes with a previous history of cataract-induced decreased vision. Phacolytic glaucoma may also develop when the lens is dislocated into the vitreous, although in these cases the intraocular inflammation is commonly less severe.

Management of phacolytic glaucoma is surgical and involves cataract extraction with intraocular lens insertion. It is quite helpful before surgery to quiet the eye and reduce IOP as much as possible. Several days' use of topical steroids, cycloplegics, aqueous suppressants, and hyperosmotic agents may be required. Miotics and prostaglandin analogs should be avoided, since they may exacerbate anterior segment inflammation.

Lens particle glaucoma

This secondary open-angle glaucoma develops when an opening in the lens capsule allows cortical material or capsular lens material to obstruct trabecular

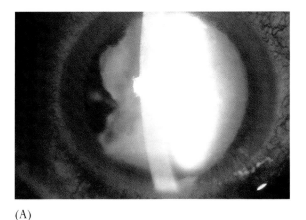

(A)

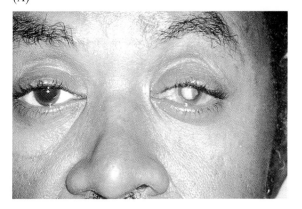

Figure 9.8A and 9.8B Lens particle glaucoma. In this patient, the surgeon attempted phacoemulsification of the lens and abandoned the surgical procedure because of technical difficulties. The patient developed increased intraocular pressure and was then referred to the glaucoma unit.

(B)

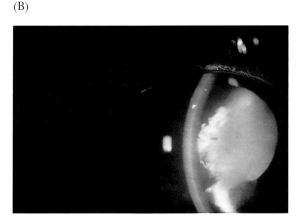

Figure 9.9 Anterior capsule rupture following a penetrating injury, leading to lens-particle glaucoma.

outflow. Lens material may gain access to the anterior chamber following incomplete removal of the lens after phacoemulsification or extracapsular cataract extraction, penetrating lens injury, Nd:YAG laser posterior capsulotomy, and even without antecedent intraocular manipulation (Figures 9.8 and 9.9).

Slit-lamp biomicroscopy shows cortical lens material circulating in the aqueous humor, lens debris deposited on the corneal endothelium, corneal edema depending upon the acuteness of the IOP rise, and significant inflammation, which may lead to a hypopyon. On gonioscopy, the angle is open, but cortical lens material usually can be identified. IOP is raised because of mechanical obstruction by the lens particles and by the inflammation associated with the process. Macrophages are also present in the anterior chamber and, in a similar manner to phacolytic glaucoma, are thought to participate minimally in the pathophysiology of the IOP increase.

Medical therapy with aqueous suppressants is indicated to reduce IOP, eventually in association with hyperosomotic agents. Cycloplegics and topical steroids are also given, whereas miotics and prostaglandin-related drugs should be avoided. If lens particle glaucoma does not respond to medical therapy or if a large amount of lens material is present, surgical removal should be prompt.

Phacoanaphylaxis

Phacoanaphylaxis can be defined as a granulomatous inflammatory response secondary to the presence of lens material. Prior sensitization to isolated lens proteins is mandatory to initiate phacoanaphylaxis, and it may occur after extracapsular cataract extraction or traumatic rupture of the lens capsule.

Although glaucoma may develop after phacoanaphylaxis, hypotony is more common. Clinical diagnosis is very difficult, and is commonly made only after enucleation and histopathology. It is characterized by a unilateral anterior uveitis that may develop days or months after lens injury.

Lens proteins are normally isolated within the lens capsule. If the capsule is ruptured, sensitization to the proteins may precipitate the granulomatous reaction. Initially, the accumulation of a polymorphonuclear infiltrate is followed by epithelioid and giant cells surrounding the damaged area. Raised IOP may be a result of several mechanisms, including trabecular obstruction by lens particle material, inflammation causing trabeculitis, or peripheral anterior synechiae.

Medical therapy with aqueous suppressants, topical and systemic steroids can be given to quiet the eye and lower the IOP before surgery. To treat this disorder, all lens particle material should be removed to stop the phacoanaphylactic response.

Phacomorphic glaucoma

Phacomorphic glaucoma is a secondary angle closure glaucoma caused by lens intumescence. Lens enlargement increases relative pupillary block and pushes the peripheral iris forward. Both mechanisms result in narrowing of the anterior chamber angle and increased IOP. The typical picture includes an asymmetrical cataract, with the contralateral eye showing a deeper anterior chamber.

Medical treatment with aqueous suppressants can be effective. Miotics are contraindicated since they increase both iridolenticular contact and the lens axial diameter, exacerbating angle closure. Since an element of pupillary block is generally present, laser iridotomy is indicated. After laser iridotomy, gonioscopy should be done to measure how wide the angle is. Major widening suggests that the pupillary component is important, whereas an angle that does not change implies that lens intumescence is the main mechanism. Subsequently, since lens intumescence is generally associated with low visual acuity, lens extraction alone may be effective in the control of IOP if peripheral anterior synechiae are not extensive.

Lens subluxation or dislocation

Lens subluxation (partial rupture of the zonules) or dislocation (complete rupture of the zonules) may cause glaucoma by several mechanisms:

a) Pupillary block by lens and/or vitreous resulting in acute or chronic angle closure.
b) Lens in the anterior chamber.
c) Lens in the vitreous causing phacolytic or lens particle glaucoma.

Several disorders are associated with ectopia lentis (Figure 9.10), such as microspherophakia (Figure 9.11), Weill–Marchesani syndrome, Marfan's syndrome (Figure 9.12)—(supero-temporal subluxation), homocystinuria (infero-nasal subluxation), simple ectopia lentis, and ectopia lentis et pupilae. Slit-lamp examination findings may vary from a discrete shift in lens position to a complete dislocation to the anterior chamber or to the vitreous. Iridodonesis and phacodonesis may also be detected. Differences in anterior chamber depths may also alert the examiner to the possibility of lens subluxation.

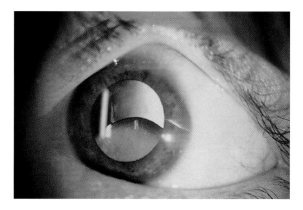

Figure 9.10 Simple ectopia lentis.

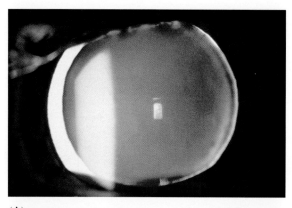

Figure 9.11
Microespherophakia, seen by trans-illumination (A), and with the lens luxated into the anterior chamber (B).

(A)

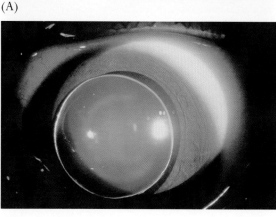

(B)

Dislocation of the lens to the anterior chamber is an emergency, since a series of complications may develop, including severe pupillary block and corneal decompensation. Medical treatment with cycloplegics with the patient in a supine position may be used when the lens is clear, to reposition it behind the iris plane, but recurrence is common. Lens extraction is the definitive treatment and is indicated in the presence of cataract, or when repositioning is unsuccessful. Pupillary block can be relieved with laser iridotomy. A lens dislocated to the vitreous may remain for many years without causing damage. Hence, conservative treatment should be encouraged, unless phacolytic glaucoma develops.

Neovascular glaucoma

Neovascular glaucoma is a secondary glaucoma caused by the presence of new vessels in the anterior chamber angle. The new vessels develop as a

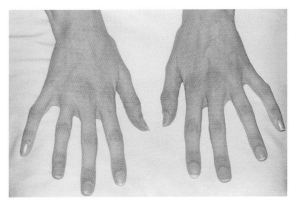

Figure 9.12
Marfan's syndrome,
with characteristic
long fingers (A), and
superiorly subluxated
lens (B).

(A)

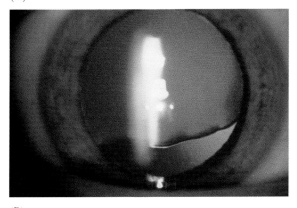

(B)

result of retinal ischemia, secondary to diabetic retinopathy, central retinal artery or vein occlusion, intraocular tumors, retinal detachment, or occlusive carotid artery disease. Ultrasound examination in patients with neovascular glaucoma and media opacities is mandatory to rule out intraocular tumors.

The first signs of incipient neovascular glaucoma are discrete tufts of new vessels in the pupillary margin (Stage I). At this stage, the angle is not yet involved. Subsequently, new vessels extend radially toward the angle (Stage II) until they finally cross over the scleral spur onto the trabecular meshowork. Occasionally, new vessels may be seen first in the anterior chamber angle. At this stage, the angle is still open, but may be crowded with new vessels, which mechanically obstruct the trabecular outflow and increase the IOP (Stage III). In a more advanced stage, the fibrovascular tissue that covers the angle pulls the peripheral iris and forms peripheral anterior synechiae that gradually lead to complete angle closure and severe IOP increase (Stage IV, Figure 9.13).

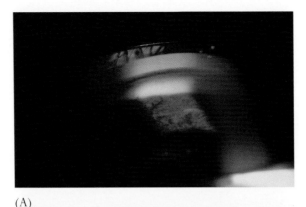

Figure 9.13A and 9.13B Neovascular glaucoma. Observe the new vessels at the peripheral iris, and a closed anterior chamber angle due to diffuse peripheral anterior synechiae.

(A)

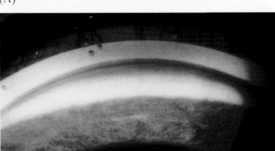

(B)

When managing neovascular glaucoma, the critical aspect is early diagnosis of patients at risk, investigating the presence of new vessels in the pupillary margin and detecting ischemic changes in the retina. Hence, patients with diabetic retinopathy or CRVO should be followed carefully to rule out rubeosis iridis. If rubeosis is detected, irrespective of the aspect of the angle, retinal panphotocoagulation must be started immediately to prevent later development of angle neovascularization and neovascular glaucoma. About 40% of patients with the ischemic type of CRVO may develop neovascular glaucoma if not treated.

Panretinal photocoagulation is the first line of therapy for most cases of neovascular glaucoma and should be done promptly at the early signs of rubeosis. In Stage III, panphotocoagulation effectively causes regression of rubeosis iridis and and new vessels in the angle, allowing an adequate IOP control without the need for surgical intervention. Aqueous suppressants, topical steroids, and cycloplegics can be used to reduce IOP and inflammation until the effect of the laser is achieved. In Stage IV, the effectiveness of panphotocoagulation in control of IOP depends on the extension of the peripheral anterior syncechiae. If the angle is circumferentially closed, panphotocoagulation is still indicated to treat retinal ischemia, but the ability to decrease IOP is limited. At this stage, medical therapy is usually unsuccessful, and filtration surgery with adjunct mitomycin C (when the rubeosis has regressed), implantation of an aqueous shunt (when the rubeosis is active), or cyclodestructive procedures (when the visual prognosis is poor) are indicated to promote adequate IOP control. In blind, painful eyes, topical steroids and atropine are often enough to reduce the pain to a tolerable level. However, cyclodestructive procedures and/or retrobulbar alcohol injection, or (rarely) enucleation are sometimes needed in painful eyes refractory to medical therapy.

Glaucoma associated with intraocular tumors

Intraocular tumors may cause glaucoma by several mechanisms:

a) Direct infiltration of the trabecular meshwork.
b) Neovascular glaucoma.
c) Secondary angle closure secondary to anterior displacement of the lens–iris diaphragm.
d) Free-floating tumor cells blocking conventional outflow (i.e. melanomalytic glaucoma).
e) Hyphema.

Tumor-induced glaucomas are usually unilateral and may be associated with several types of tumors, mainly uveal melanomas, uveal metastasis, and retinoblastoma. However, benign tumors, such as iris melanocytomas and medulloepitheliomas, can also cause glaucoma. Lymphoid tumors and leukemias may infiltrate the uveal tract and retina, resulting in blockage of aqueous outflow. Retinoblastoma, the most common malignancy of childhood, is associated with glaucoma in about 15% of cases.

Identifying the tumor as the cause of glaucoma is essential in establishing the best treatment strategy (Figure 9.14). Adequate gonioscopy, indirect ophthal-

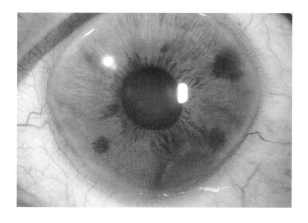

Figure 9.14 Iris melanoma in a patient with secondary elevation of intraocular pressure. The lesion had invaded the adjacent anterior chamber angle, and there was increased pigmentation in the trabecular meshwork.

moscopy, and ultrasound examination may disclose this uncommon but potentially life-threatening cause of glaucoma. Eyes with malignant tumors should not undergo filtration surgery. Cyclodestructive procedures or a retrobulbar alcohol injection should be considered in a painful eye in which the tumor cannot be treated.

Glaucoma secondary to increased episcleral venous pressure

The modified Goldmann equation, $Po = F/C + Pev$ (where Po = intraocular pressure, F = aqueous production, C = outflow facility and Pev = episcleral venous pressure) illustrates the direct association between episcleral venous pressure and intraocular pressure. Hence, increasing the episcleral venous pressures (whose normal values range from 9 to 10 mmHg) leads to an increase in intraocular pressure.

Glaucoma may be caused by any disorder that causes compression of the venous drainage of the eye, especially the superior ophthalmic vein. Compression may be caused by retrobulbar tumors, thyroid ophthalmopathy, thrombosis of the cavernous sinus or the superior ophthalmic vein, jugular vein obstruction, and superior vena cava syndrome. Increased episcleral venous pressure may also be a consequence of arteriovenous anomalies such as carotid cavernous fistulas (Figure 9.15), or congenital abnormalities such as orbital varices. Episcleral hemangiomas seen in Sturge–Weber syndrome may also promote high episcleral venous pressure (Figure 9.16). Finally, idiopathic cases of increased episcleral venous pressure have been described (Figure 9.17).

Patients with raised episcleral venous pressure show dilated, tortuous episcleral veins. The angle is typically open, eventually allowing the visualization of blood in Schlemm's canal. The glaucoma may be unilateral (when secondary to Sturge–Weber syndrome or orbital varices) or bilateral when the venous

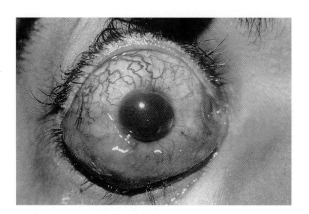

Figure 9.15
Dilated, tortuous episcleral vessels, conjunctival chemosis and proptosis in a patient with a direct carotid cavernous fistula.

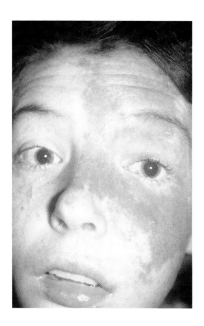

Figure 9.16 Sturge–Weber syndrome. Episcleral hemangiomas are associated with high episcleral venous pressure.

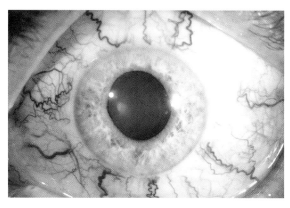

Figure 9.17
Idiopathic increased episcleral venous pressure, with prominent tortuous episcleral vessels.

compression is localized in the neck (i.e. superior vena cava syndrome). Carotid cavernous fistulas may result in unilateral or bilateral glaucoma, since there is a communication between the sinuses.

If possible, treatment of glaucoma should be directed to the cause of raised episcleral venous pressure. When this strategy is impossible or unsuccessful, medical therapy with aqueous suppressants and prostaglandin-related drugs should be commenced. Although aqueous suppressants will not decrease IOP below the episcleral venous pressure, prostaglandin-related drugs should be effective in doing so since they increase uveoscleral outflow. Laser trabeculoplasty is generally not effective. On the other hand, filtration surgery can be attempted, but is associated with a higher rate of complications, including

135

choroidal effusions and suprachoroidal hemorrhage. Tight closure of the scleral flap combined with prophylactic sclerostomies may help reduce postoperative complications.

Inflammatory glaucomas

Intraocular inflammation alters the dynamics of aqueous humor, and may cause raised or reduced IOP. The latter is associated with decreased aqueous humor production and increased uveoscleral outflow. On the other hand, inflammatory glaucoma may be explained by a variety of mechanisms, including:

a) Obstruction of the trabecular meshwork by inflammatory cells and protein.
b) Trabeculitis (inflammation of the trabecular meshwork itself).
c) Formation of peripheral anterior synechiae.
d) Posterior synechiae leading to pupillary block (Figure 9.18).
e) Iris neovascularization and neovascular glaucoma.
f) Anterior rotation of the lens–iris diaphragm.

All forms of uveitis may result in glaucoma through one or more of the mechanisms above. In Fuch's heterochromic cyclitis (Figure 9.19), the affected eye shows a triad consisting of heterochromia (lighter iris color than the contralateral eye), uveitis (low grade, usually symptom-free), and cataract. Keratic precipitates are fine, colorless, star-shaped, and scattered over the endothelium. Open-angle glaucoma may develop in later stages in 25% of cases. Patients may have fine neovascularization of the iris and the anterior chamber angle, which may bleed. Both eyes are affected in about 10% of patients.

Glaucomatocyclitic crisis, also known as Posner–Schlossman syndrome, is characterized by recurrent episodes of unilateral anterior uveitis and raised IOP. Symptoms include slight ocular discomfort, halos and blurred vision. As

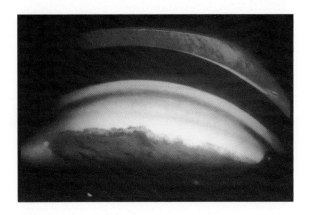

Figure 9.18
Extensive peripheral anterior synechiae in a patient with inflammatory glaucoma.

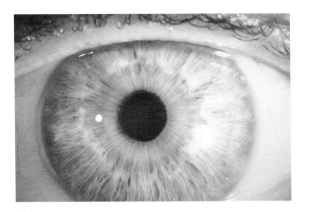

(A)

Figure 9.19
Patient with Fuch's heterochromic cyclitis. The normal eye (A) has a darker iris color than the affected eye (B). Fine neovascularization of the iris (B) and the anterior chamber angle (C) is noted.

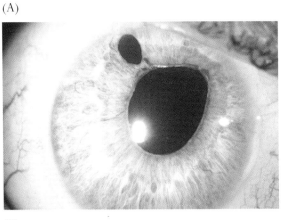

(B)

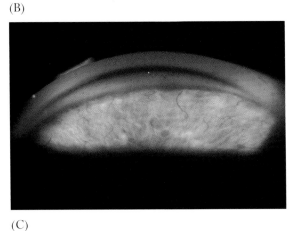

(C)

heterochromic cyclitis, it occurs in young to middle-aged adults. Slit-lamp examination discloses a few fine nonpigmented keratic precipitates in an eye with very high IOP and mild anterior chamber reaction. The attack usually

137

subsides in between 1 and 3 weeks. Patients may develop chronically raised IOPs leading to optic nerve and visual field damage.

Treatment of inflammatory glaucoma includes topical and systemic steroids, cycloplegics, and antiglaucoma medications. Steroids can also contribute to IOP increase. In uveitic eyes with raised IOP, open angle and on steroid therapy, it may be difficult to know whether the IOP increase was secondary to the inflammatory condition or steroid response. In this situation, if the inflammation damages the eye, steroids are continued to decrease the inflammation and the IOP treated as necessary to prevent optic nerve injury. Without losing control of the inflammation, if possible, the steroids should be reduced or replaced by a nonsteroidal antiinflammatory or a steroid less likely to increase IOP.

Cycloplegics prevent the formation of a miotic secluded pupil, increase uveoscleral outflow, stabilize the blood–aqueous barrier, and relieve pain from ciliary spasm. Aqueous suppressants are effective, whereas miotics and prostaglandin-related drugs should be avoided because they worsen the breakdown in the blood–aqueous barrier. Laser trabeculoplasty is not successful in control of IOP, and may actually increase inflammation. Filtering surgery without antimetabolites is associated with poor success rates. Hence, intraoperative mitomycin C or 5-FU is mandatory to increase the chances of success. Many glaucoma specialists prefer aqueous shunts for patients with chronic or recurrent inflammation, whereas cyclodestructive procedures are reserved for refractory cases.

Ghost-cell glaucoma

Ghost-cell glaucoma is caused by the obstruction of the trabecular meshwork by degenerated red blood cells. These ghost cells are spherical red blood cells that have lost most of their intracellular hemoglobin. The remaining hemoglobin is denatured and contained in characteristic Heinz bodies (Figure 9.20). Ghost cells are less pliable than biconcave red blood cells, which limits their passage through the intertrabecular spaces. Ghost cells are formed in the vitreous some weeks after a vitreous hemorrhage. The degenerated cells migrate to the anterior chamber through a defect in the vitreous face and obstruct trabecular outflow. Post-traumatic and post-surgical hyphemas may disperse to the vitreous, allowing the formation of ghost cells, which can then return to the anterior chamber and cause raised IOP.

Slit-lamp examination discloses khaki-colored cells in the anterior chamber (which may form a tan pseudohypopion), anterior vitreous, and trabecular meshwork. Aqueous suppressants are usually effective in lowering IOP. Miotics and argon laser trabeculoplasty are not good options. Performing two paracenteses and washing out the anterior chamber with balanced salt solution removes the ghost cells and may control IOP. However, when there is a large source of

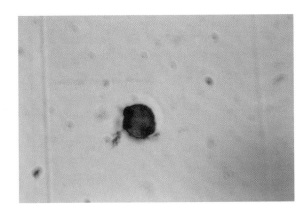

Figure 9.20 Ghost cell with Heinz bodies obtained from a paracentesis (magnification, ×100).

degenerated cells in the vitreous, anterior chamber lavage results in a transitory reduction of IOP, and pars plana vitrectomy is then indicated.

Glaucomas associated with ocular surgery

Glaucoma may develop after any intraocular surgery, more often by compromising trabecular outflow. Although vitreoretinal surgery and penetrating keratoplasty may result in postoperative raised IOP, we will focus on the secondary glaucomas associated with aphakia or caused by epithelial downgrowth or fibrous ingrowth.

Glaucoma in aphakia and pseudophakia

The prevalence of glaucoma after cataract surgery has decreased over the years owing to a marked improvement in surgical techniques. A high prevalence (between 5% and 12%) was observed after intracapsular cataract extraction or complicated cataract extraction (42%). Glaucoma is also more common with use of AC IOLs (5.5–6.3%) or iris-fixated lenses (3.9–4.3%) than PC IOLs (1.6–3.5%). Eyes with preexisting glaucoma have a higher risk of developing IOP spikes after cataract surgery, which stimulates the indication of combined cataract–glaucoma surgery in patients with advanced glaucomatous damage (see Chapter 13).

IOP increase may develop after uncomplicated or complicated cataract surgery in the early or late postoperative periods and may be precipitated by one or more of the following mechanisms:

a) Preexisting glaucoma.
b) Hyphema.

139

c) Viscoelastic material.
d) Trabecular edema.
e) Inflammation.
f) Vitreous in the anterior chamber.
g) Lens-particle glaucoma.
h) Corticosteroid-induced glaucoma.
i) Ghost-cell glaucoma.
j) Pupillary block (by posterior synechiae, gas bubble, vitreous, silicone oil).
k) Malignant glaucoma.
l) Epithelial ingrowth.

Identifying the mechanism(s) associated with raised IOP is essential in determining treatment strategy. Helpful clues include the verification of anterior chamber depth and inflammation, examination of the angle and the optic nerve head. The reader should refer to each session dealing with the mechanisms above in order to obtain guidelines to treatment.

Epithelial downgrowth and fibrous ingrowth

Epithelial downgrowth refers to the presence of epithelium in the anterior chamber. Invasion of epithelium (mainly from the conjunctiva) occurs through an imperfectly healed wound. Fortunately, the prevalence has decreased from 17–26% in the older literature to 0.08% over the past decade. Improvement in microsurgical techniques, especially in wound closure, may explain the marked decrease. Slit-lamp examination discloses an injected eye with a wound gape (positive Seidel test) early in the disease, which allows epithelial cells to gain access to the anterior chamber. The cornea is edematous and usually shows a posterior membrane demarcated by a gray line, which represents the epithelial sheet (Figure 9.21). The epithelial sheet grows over the iris and ciliary body, leading to mechanical obstruction of the angle, formation of peripheral anterior synechiae, and glaucoma (reported in 43% of cases). Argon laser photocoagulation of the iris surface (100–200 mW for 0.1 sec over a 200 micron spot size) produces a fluffy white lesion in areas covered by abnormal epithelium, and is used to demarcate the extension of iris involvement (Figure 9.22). Medical treatment of glaucoma secondary to epithelial downgrowth is usually ineffective. Surgical treatment includes closure of the fistula if it still exists and destruction with laser or extirpation of the involved tissue (iris, ciliary body and vitreous), followed by transcorneal and transscleral cryotherapy to devitalize the epithelium on the posterior surface of the cornea, the angle and the ciliary body. Visual acuity can be improved with penetrating keratoplasty, and IOP

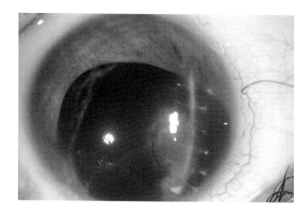

Figure 9.21
Epithelial downgrowth
secondary to a
penetrating ocular
injury. Observe the
retrocorneal grayish
plaque.

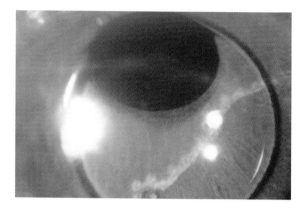

Figure 9.22
Epithelial
downgrowth. Argon
laser photocoagulation
is used to demarcate
the extension of iris
involvement. The
argon laser produces a
fluffy white lesion in
areas covered by
abnormal epithelium.

control is better obtained with aqueous shunts. If the visual potential does not justify excision of the membrane, an aqueous shunt and topical steroid and atropine usually results in a comfortable eye with controlled IOP.

Fibrous ingrowth refers to the development of a retrocorneal membrane formed by fibrocellular proliferative tissue, and is more common after penetrating keratoplasty. It behaves less aggressively than epithelial downgrowth and is frequently self-limited. Fibrous ingrowth is also associated with poor wound closure and hypotony, and is characterized by a fibrous membrane with a gray-white color and overlying corneal edema. Glaucoma may develop as a consequence of the obstruction of angle structures, peripheral anterior synechiae, or recurrent bleeding. Medical management is directed to control inflammation and IOP. Depending on the severity of fibrous ingrowth and the visual prognosis, trabeculectomy with adjunct mitomycin C, aqueous shunt implantation, or a cyclodestructive procedure may be indicated.

141

Iridocorneal endothelial syndrome

Iridocorneal endothelial syndrome (ICE) is characterized by a primary abnormality of the corneal endothelium associated with variable degrees of corneal edema, iris atrophy, and progressive angle closure leading to glaucoma. This

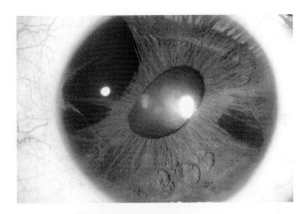

Figure 9.23
Essential iris atrophy – progression of iris changes with marked iris atrophy over a follow-up of ten years (A–C).

(A)

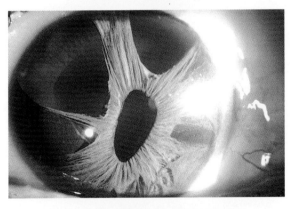

(B)

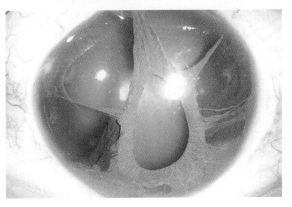

(C)

condition is almost always unilateral and preferentially affects women in the third to fifth decades. There are three different clinical presentations:

a) Progressive or essential iris atrophy – This variation is characterized by predominance of the iris changes with marked iris atrophy, corectopia, ectropion uveae, and hole formation (Figure 9.23). The pupil is generally distorted toward the quadrant with the most prominent area of peripheral anterior synechiae. Holes may also develop as a consequence of traction (opposite to the quadrant with PAS), or ischemia (melting holes, observed in areas with no evidence of traction).
b) Chandler's syndrome (Figure 9.24) – Changes in the cornea are more prominent, whereas iris abnormalities are mild and glaucoma less common.
c) Cogan–Reese syndrome (Figure 9.25) – Pigmented, pedunculated iris nodules are typical, and may be associated with the previously described corneal and iris changes.

Common features in all clinical presentations include a corneal–endothelial change characterized by a fine hammered silver appearance at slit lamp biomicroscopy. Specular microscopy discloses pleomorphism, loss of the hexagonal

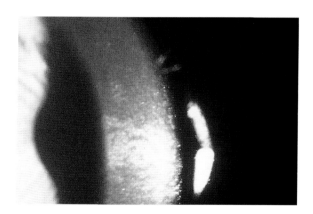

Figure 9.24
Chandler's syndrome, with characteristic 'hammered silver appearance' of the endothelium.

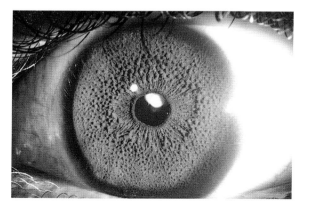

Figure 9.25
Cogan–Reese syndrome. Pigmented iris nodules covering the surface of the iris.

143

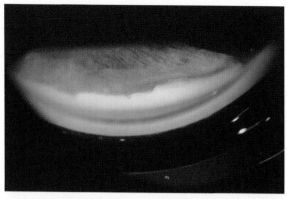

Figure 9.26A and 9.26B: Characteristic gonioscopic changes of eyes with iridocorneal endothelial syndrome: there are very anterior and irregular peripheral anterior synechiae.

(A)

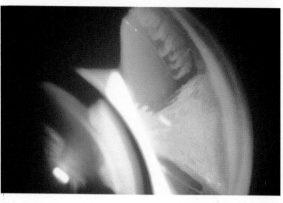

(B)

margins and dark areas within the cells. Gonioscopy reveals peripheral anterior synechiae extending anterior to Schwalbe's line (Figure 9.26). Glaucoma develops in 50% of patients with ICE syndrome, and tends to be more severe with progressive iris atrophy and Cogan–Reese syndrome. Obstruction of the trabecular meshwork may occur as a result of synechial angle closure or from a cellular membrane formed by a single layer of endothelial cells and a Descemet-like membrane extending posteriorly from the peripheral cornea.

The precise pathogenesis of ICE syndrome is unclear. It may be a result of an inflammatory condition. In fact, two independent investigators suggested an association with the Epstein–Barr and the herpes simplex viruses. It is generally accepted, however, that changes in the corneal endothelium are the basis of all other clinical findings.

Adequate IOP control in patients with ICE syndrome may be achieved in the early stages with aqueous suppressants. Lowering IOP may help control the corneal edema. Laser trabeculoplasty is unsuccessful, and filtering surgery often

144

fails due to obstruction of the internal sclerostomy by the cellular membrane. In this case, it is possible to re-open the fistula at least for a short while with Nd:YAG laser applications. In cases of severe corneal edema, penetrating kerato-plasty is considered after the glaucoma has been controlled.

Suggested reading

Becker B. Intraocular pressure reponse to topical corticosteroids. *Invest Ophthalmol* 1965;**4**:198–202.

Brown GC, Magargal LE, Schachat A et al. Neovascular glaucoma: etiologic considerations. *Ophthalmology* 1984;**91**:315–20.

Campbell DG, Simons RJ, Grant WM. Ghost cells as a cause of glaucoma. *Am J Ophthalmol* 1976;**81**:441–5.

Costa VP, Katz LJ, Cohen EJ, Raber IM. Glaucoma associated with epithelial downgrowth controlled with Molteno tube shunts. *Ophthalm Surg* 1992;**23**:797–800.

Epstein DL, Jedziniak JA, Grant WM. Obstruction of aqueous outflow by lens particles and by heavy molecular weight soluble lens proteins. *Invest Ophthalmol Vis Sci* 1978;**17**:272–7.

Farrar SM, Shields MB. Current concepts in pigmentary glaucoma. *Surv Ophthalmol* 1993;**37**:233–52.

Fiore PM, Latina MA, Shingleton BJ et al. The dural shunt syndrome. I. Management of glaucoma. *Ophthalmology* 1990;**97**:56–61.

Gross RL, Feldman RM, Spaeth GL et al. Surgical therapy of chronic glaucoma in aphakia and pseudophakia. *Ophthalmology* 1988;**95**:1195–200.

Iwach AG, Hoskins HD, Hetherington J et al. Analysis of surgical and medical management of glaucoma in Sturge–Weber syndrome. *Ophthalmology* 1990;**97**:904–9.

Kaufman JH, Tolpin DW. Glaucoma after traumatic angle recession. *Am J Ophthalmol* 1974;**78**:648–53.

Krupin T, Feitl ME, Karalekas D. Glaucoma associated with uveitis. In: Ritch R, Shields MB, Krupin T (eds). *The Glaucomas*, 2nd edition. St Louis: CV Mosby Co, 1996; 1225–58.

Myers J, Katz LJ. Secondary open-angle glaucomas. In: Choplin NT, Lundy DC (eds). *Atlas of glaucoma*. London: Martin Dunitz, 1998; 115–32.

Richter CU. Lens-induced open-angle glaucoma. In: Ritch R, Shields MB, Krupin T (eds). *The Glaucomas*, 2nd edition. St Louis: CV Mosby Co, 1996; 1023–31.

Ritch R. Exfoliation Syndrome. In: Ritch R, Shields MB, Krupin T (eds). *The Glaucomas*, 2nd edition. St Louis: CV Mosby Co, 1996; 993–1022.

Shields CL, Shields JA, Shields MB, Augsburger JJ. Prevalence and mechanisms of intraocular pressure elevation in eyes with intraocular tumors. *Ophthalmology* 1987;**94**:839–44.

Shields MB. Progressive essential iris atrophy, Chandler's syndrome, and the iris–nevus (Cogan–Reese) syndrome: a spectrum of disease. *Surv Ophthalmol* 1979;**24**:3–19.

Spaeth GL, Rodrigues MM, Weinreb S. Steroid-induced glaucoma. A. Persistent elevation of intraocular pressure. B. Histopathologic aspects. *Trans Am Ophthalmol Soc* 1977;**75**:353–65.

Wand M, Dueker DK, Aiello LM, Grant WM. Effects of panretinal photocoagulation on rubeosis iridis, angle neovascularization, and neovascular glaucoma. *Am J Ophthalmol* 1978;**86**:332–7.

10. PEDIATRIC GLAUCOMA AND GLAUCOMA ASSOCIATED WITH DEVELOPMENTAL DISORDERS

Augusto Azuara-Blanco, Richard P Wilson, and Vital P Costa

Introduction

Glaucoma in children is rare, about 1 in 10 000 births. A general ophthalmologist will probably see only one case of glaucoma in children every 5 years. However, severe visual disability is a common consequence of this disorder. Optic nerve damage, corneal scarring and amblyopia are the most common causes of visual loss. Early diagnosis and appropriate therapy can make a huge difference in the visual outcome of these patients.

Glaucoma in children can be classified into three groups: (I) *primary congenital glaucoma*, due to an isolated congenital abnormality of the trabecular meshwork; (II) *developmental glaucoma*, related to a congenital anomaly of the anterior segment associated with other ocular or systemic abnormalities; and (III) *acquired childhood glaucoma*, in which the obstruction to outflow is related to other acquired events such as inflammation or the use of topical steroids.

Primary congenital glaucoma

Primary congenital glaucoma is the most common form of glaucoma in children. It usually appears shortly after birth and, in most cases, within the first year of life. It is bilateral in 70% of patients. Males are more commonly affected than females (3:2 ratio). Although autosomal recessive inheritance is detected in 10% of patients, most cases have a multifactorial inheritance. Mutations in the CYP1B1 gene, located in chromosome 2p21, are thought to be responsible for 85–90% of the familial cases.

Clinical features and diagnosis

1. *When glaucoma appears in the first year of life*, symptoms of epiphora, photophobia (due to corneal edema) and blepharospasm are typical (Table 10.1). Since the eye is elastic, stretching and enlargement of the cornea and the globe are noted (Figure 10.1). Untreated eyes may become very large or 'buphthalmic' (cow's eye).

Table 10.1 Differential diagnosis of congenital glaucoma in children

	Excessive tearing	Large cornea	Tears in Descemet's membrane	Corneal opacity	Other findings
Glaucoma	+	+	+ (concentric to limbus, horizontal)	+/–	Photophobia Disc cupping High IOP Gonioscopic findings
Nasolacrimal duct obstruction	+	–	–	–	Fullness of lacrimal sac Purulent discharge
Megalocornea	–	+	–	–	Enlarged anterior segment
Birth trauma	–	–	+ (vertical)	+/-	

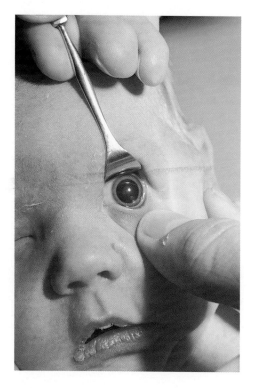

Figure 10.1 External examination of patient with congenital glaucoma and enlarged globe.

Infants require general anesthesia for a reliable examination. Tonometry, measurement of the corneal diameter and axial length, examination of the cornea and anterior chamber (best done with a portable slit-lamp), gonioscopy, and ophthalmoscopy are important tools for diagnosing and monitoring glaucoma in children.

Most anesthetics lower the intraocular pressure (IOP), with the exception of ketamine. IOP should be measured as soon as possible after induction of anesthesia to obtain reliable measurements. Tonometry should be done with at least two different systems (e.g. applanation tonometry and Tonopen). The normal IOP in infants is lower than that of adults. An IOP of 20 mmHg or more is diagnostic, and IOPs above 15 mmHg are suspicious.

Measurement of the horizontal corneal diameter with calipers may be a more reliable guide than the vertical diameter or the axial length in the assessment of glaucoma in infants. The normal horizontal corneal diameter varies between 10–10.5 mm in neonates, and 11–11.5 mm at 1 year of age. Measurements greater than 12 mm during the first year of life are highly suggestive of glaucoma. Axial length determination with A-scan ultrasound is another useful tool to monitor glaucoma.

The corneal stroma may become edematous and hazy as a direct result of raised IOP. The epithelium is edematous and prone to erosions and scarring. Tears in Descemet's membrane oriented horizontally or concentric to the limbus (Haab's striae) are common and usually associated with stromal edema (Figures 10.2 and 10.3). They should be differentiated from vertical central tears in Descemet's membrane related to birth trauma. The corneal edema and haziness can disappear with normalization of the IOP, but in more advanced cases permanent corneal opacity may occur.

In patients with isolated trabeculodysgenesis (the most common form), the anterior chamber is deep, and the iris and the cornea have a normal appearance. Other patients may have iris and/or corneal anomalies (e.g. iris stromal defects or anomalous iris vessels). Lens subluxation may occur in advanced cases.

Gonioscopy should be done if corneal clarity allows. A direct goniolens (e.g. infant Koeppe lens) and an operating microscope are ideal. In a normal infant, the iris inserts flatly into the ciliary body, and the normal trabecular meshwork appears as a smooth homogeneous membrane. In primary congenital glaucoma, the iris insertion is anterior, forming a scalloped line.

Ophthalmoscopy and assessment of the optic nerve are essential to diagnose and monitor glaucoma in children. Examination by direct ophthalmoscopy is facilitated by the use of a Koeppe lens or a contact lens used for vitrectomy surgery. Normal infants have a smaller C/D ratio than adults (most commonly C/D ratio < 0.3). In children with glaucoma the optic cup is larger and typically concentric, with a preferential loss in the vertical poles in advanced cases. Lowering the IOP in children with glaucoma is commonly associated with reversal of optic disc cupping.

149

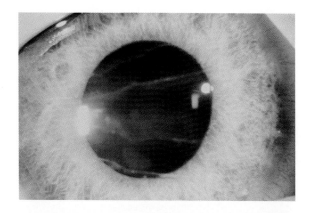

Figure 10.2 Haab's striae in congenital glaucoma. Note typical pattern of rail-like refractile material at the level of Descemet's membrane with a horizontal orientation.

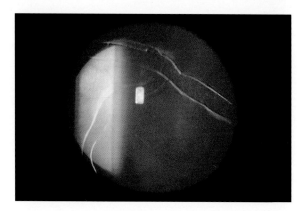

Figure 10.3 Haab's striae are easily seen with pupil dilated, using the red reflex.

2. *When glaucoma appears in older children (up to 3 years of age)*, progressive enlargement of the globe and myopia may be indicative of uncontrolled glaucoma. After 3 years of age, the eye no longer expands in response to raised IOP.

3. *Juvenile glaucoma* refers to all forms of open-angle glaucoma diagnosed between the ages of 3 years and adulthood.

Treatment

Congenital glaucoma is managed surgically. Medical therapy is used before surgery or when repeated surgical procedures have failed. Success of surgical treatments is related to the severity and duration of the glaucoma. The worst prognosis occurs in infants with raised pressures and cloudy corneas at birth. The best prognosis is seen in infants with isolated trabeculodysgenesis operated between the second and eighth months of life.

Goniotomy and *trabeculotomy* (see Chapter 13) are very effective operations in primary congenital glaucoma due to trabeculodysgenesis and they produce similar results. Success rates range from 60% to 90%, although in one-third to one-half of the eyes the procedure must be repeated. Success rates decrease in eyes with iris and/or corneal anomalies. Goniotomy has the advantage of preserving the conjunctiva for possible future filtering procedures. However, goniotomy cannot be done in cases of corneal clouding, and trabeculotomy is preferred to trabeculectomy.

If *goniotomy* and *trabeculotomy* are unsuccessful, trabeculectomy with mild mitomycin-C is recommended. Trabeculectomy, with or without mitomycin-C, can be combined with trabeculotomy. Because of the complications of late bleb leak and endophthalmitis, aqueous shunts are an alternative to trabeculectomy in the young. Shunts are always used before cyclodestructive procedures, which are the final option.

Even when the IOP is well controlled, a significant number of children never achieve good vision. The most common cause of poor vision is amblyopia related to anisometropia. Therefore, cycloplegic refraction is essential to prevent amblyopia. Occasionally, the corneal opacity may be permanent and penetrating keratoplasty may be indicated.

Glaucoma associated with developmental disorders

Aniridia

Aniridia is a hereditary bilateral congenital disorder characterized by the partial or total absence of iris (Figure 10.4). It is transmitted as an autosomal dominant trait in two-thirds of cases. A third of cases are sporadic and can be associated with Wilms' tumor (in 20% of patients). An autosomal recessive mode of inheritance has also been described.

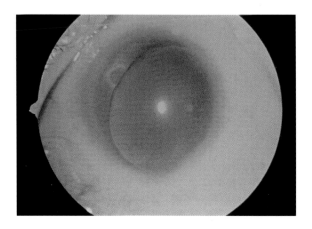

Figure 10.4 Infant with aniridia and subluxated lens.

151

Other common ocular abnormalities include limbal stem cell deficiency and corneal pannus, cataracts (very common after the third decade of life), ectopia lentis, and foveal hypoplasia with reduced vision and nystagmus. Glaucoma occurs in 50–75% of patients with aniridia, usually in late childhood, and is caused by progressive angle closure by the iris remnants. Possible systemic abnormalities include genitourinary abnormalities and mental retardation.

Medical treatment is the initial line of therapy. Although goniotomy and trabeculotomy can be considered in young children, filtering surgery is usually the best surgical approach.

Axenfeld–Rieger syndrome

Axenfeld–Rieger syndrome is a bilateral developmental disorder, with an autosomal dominant inheritance, a high incidence of associated glaucoma (more than 50%) and systemic developmental defects. There is no differentiation by sex, and most cases are diagnosed during childhood.

Three clinical variations have been described:

'*Axenfeld's anomaly*' consists of a thickened and anteriorly displaced Schwalbe's line, or posterior embryotoxon (seen on slit-lamp examination as a white line on the posterior cornea near the limbus, Figure 10.5) with abundant anterior strands of uveal tissue attached to Schwalbe's line (Figure 10.6). These strands bridge the anterior chamber angle from the peripheral iris to the prominent ridge, and beyond these strands the trabecular meshwork is visible. The number and size of iris strands is highly variable, and is not related to the presence of glaucoma. An isolated posterior embryotoxon occurs in 10% of the general population and is not associated with glaucoma or systemic anomalies.

'*Rieger's anomaly*' designates Axenfeld's anomaly plus changes in the iris (from mild iris thinning to marked atrophy with polycoria (more than one pupil), corectopia, and ectopia uveae). Many other ocular anomalies have been reported.

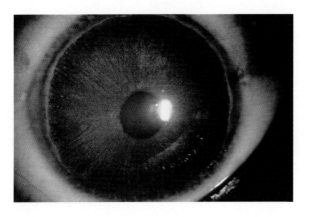

Figure 10.5
Axenfeld anomaly with posterior embriotoxon.

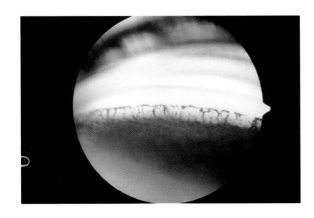

Figure 10.6
Gonioscopic view of numerous iris strands characteristic of Axenfeld–Rieger syndrome.

'*Rieger's syndrome*' consists of ocular anomalies plus systemic developmental defects, most commonly dental (microdontia, hypodontia) and facial anomalies (maxillary hypoplasia, flattening of midface, receding upper lip and prominent lower lip). Anomalies of the pituitary gland region have been reported in several patients. Other neurological, dermatological and skeletal disorders have been described.

Goniosurgery is not as successful as in eyes with primary congenital glaucoma. Trabeculectomy, whether associated with trabeculotomy or not, with or without mitomycin-C, may be indicated if medical therapy is unsuccessful.

Peters' anomaly

Peters' anomaly is a sporadic anomaly present at birth, characterized by a central defect in Descemet's membrane and corneal endothelium with stromal thinning (posterior keratoconus) and opacification. Iris adhesions typically extend to the borders of the corneal defect. 80% percent of cases are bilateral.

There are different degrees of adhesions of the lens and the iris to the cornea, and three types of Peters' anomaly have been differentiated: I. no keratolenticular contact or cataract; II. keratolenticular contact or cataract (Figures 10.7 and 10.8); III. with peripheral anomalies typical of Axenfeld–Rieger syndrome.

About 50% of patients with Peters' anomaly will develop glaucoma, which usually requires surgical intervention (trabeculectomy). Penetrating keratoplasty is often needed, although the outcome is poor.

Sturge–Weber syndrome

Sturge–Weber syndrome is characterized by a facial hemangioma in the distribution of the trigeminal nerve, which may be associated with meningeal

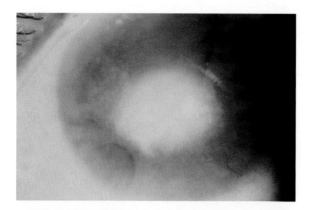

Figure 10.7 Peter's anomaly with central opacity.

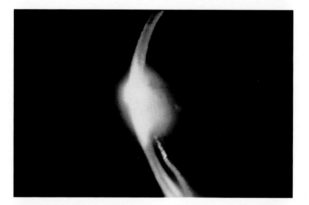

Figure 10.8 Slit-lamp view of Peters' anomaly with lens-corneal adhesions and shallow anterior chamber.

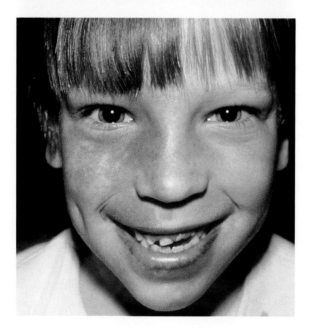

Figure 10.9 Sturge–Weber syndrome. There is extensive facial hemangioma involving the trigeminal nerve.

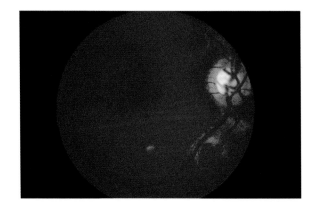

Figure 10.10
Choroidal
hemangioma in a
patient with
Sturge–Weber
syndrome. Note the
'tomato catsup'
appearance of the
fundus.

hemangiomas that can cause seizures (Figure 10.9). The disease is usually unilateral. Ocular hemangiomas can affect the conjunctiva, episcleral vessels, iris, angle, choroid or retina (Figure 10.10). Glaucoma is common when the hemangioma involves the lid or the conjunctiva, and is explained by two different mechanisms: abnormal development of the trabecular meshwork; and raised episcleral venous pressure.

Medical treatment can be attempted. Goniotomy and trabeculotomy are reasonably successful in infants who typically have a goniodysgenesis, but poor in older children. Infants and young children who do well with goniotomy or trabeculotomy usually require a trabeculectomy at 7 to 10 years of age. Combined trabeculotomy and trabeculectomy is recommended by several authors for children with glaucoma associated with the Sturge–Weber syndrome. However, filtration surgery is frequently complicated by choroidal effusions and there is an increased risk of intra- and postoperative suprachoroidal hemorrhage. Prophylactic sclerostomies may be considered at the time of filtering surgery, and intraoperative and postoperative hypotony should be avoided.

Nanophthalmos

This rare anomaly is characterized by a small eye (axial length < 20 mm), reduced corneal diameter, high lens/eye volume ratio, shallow anterior chamber and narrow anterior chamber angle. These eyes are highly hyperopic and develop angle closure glaucoma in the fourth to sixth decades of life. Severe uveal effusions and nonrhegmatogenous retinal detachment are likely after intraocular surgery. These complications are secondary to reduced uveoscleral outflow, which is thought to be related to an abnormally thick sclera.

Laser iridotomy and peripheral iridoplasty are the initial procedures of choice. If filtration surgery is needed, scleral windows (dissecting areas of sclera to two-thirds thickness) and/or full-thickness sclerostomies should be done before opening the globe to prevent the accumulation of fluid in the suprachoroidal space.

Glaucoma after congenital cataract surgery

Cataracts in children (Figure 10.11) can be treated by lens aspiration with or without posterior capsulotomy and possible anterior vitrectomy. Intraocular lenses may be inserted in the posterior chamber. Glaucoma after cataract surgery in children is a common and severe complication but the cause of the glaucoma is controversial. It is possible that the trabecular meshwork is damaged by lens remnants and inflammation. Pupillary block and angle closure is an uncommon cause, since the use of vitreous cutting instruments allows a more complete removal of vitreous and lens tissue. Finally, it is suggested that some of these patients may already have an abnormal anterior chamber angle at birth.

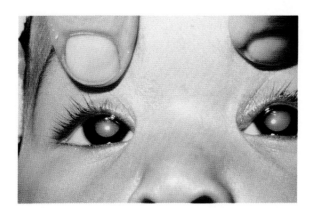

Figure 10.11
Bilateral congenital cataract.

Glaucoma in aphakic children is a very challenging problem. Goniosurgery is not useful, and the outcome of trabeculectomy with mitomycin-C is usually poor. Glaucoma drainage devices and cyclodestructive procedures are often needed.

Suggested reading

Anderson DR. The development of the trabecular meshwork and its abnormality in primary infantile glaucoma. *Trans Am Ophthalmol Soc* 1981;**79**:461.

Azuara-Blanco A, Spaeth GL, Araujo SV et al. Ultrasound biomicroscopy in infantile glaucoma. *Ophthalmology* 1997;**104**:1116.

Azuara-Blanco A, Wilson RP, Spaeth GL et al. Filtration procedures supplemented with mitomycin C in the management of childhood glaucoma. *Br J Ophthalmol* 1999;**83**:151.

Beauchamp GR, Parks MM. Filtering surgery in children. Barriers to success. *Ophthalmology* 1979;**86**:170.

DeLuise VP, Anderson DR. Primary infantile glaucoma (congenital glaucoma). *Surv Ophthalmol* 1983;**28**:1.

Hill RA, Heuer DK, Baerveldt G et al. Molteno implantation for glaucoma in young patients. *Ophthalmology* 1991;**98**:1042.

Hodapp E, Heuer DK. A simple technique for goniotomy. *Am J Ophthalmol* 1986;**102**:537.

Hoskins DH, Shaffer RN, Hetherington J. Goniotomy vs. trabeculotomy. *J Pediatric Ophthalmol Strab* 1984;**21**:153.

Netland PA, Walton DS. Glaucoma drainage implants in pediatric patients. *Ophthalmic Surg* 1993;**24**:723.

Quigley HA. Childhood glaucoma. Results with trabeculotomy and study of reversible cupping. *Ophthalmology* 1982;**89**:219.

Walton DS. Primary congenital open angle glaucoma. A study of the anterior segment abnormalities. *Trans Am Ophthalmol Soc* 1979;**77**:746.

SECTION III
TREATMENT

11. MEDICAL THERAPY

Vital P Costa, Richard P Wilson, and Augusto Azuara-Blanco

Medical therapy

The aim of glaucoma treatment is to preserve patients' sight, while maintaining as much as possible their quality of life. Although several mechanisms have been proposed to explain the loss of retinal ganglion cells that characterizes glaucoma, lowering the intraocular pressure (IOP) is the only scientifically proven strategy that results in stabilization of the disease. Studies investigating the repercussion of blood flow improvement and neuroprotection on the natural history of the disease are being undertaken, but long-term follow-up is needed before we can confirm their effectiveness in the treatment of glaucoma. Hence, this chapter will focus on the hypotensive efficacy and safety of several drugs currently used to treat glaucoma.

General guidelines

There are some guidelines that need to be followed whenever a patient is started on medical therapy. The first one has to do with uniocular therapeutic trials. It is almost always beneficial to do a one-eyed therapeutic trial, i.e. to test the effect of a drug in only one eye, which will allow the comparison with the untreated, contralateral eye. Second, substituting drugs is always preferable to adding drugs, especially now that market availability of drugs has increased. When adding medications, it is helpful to try to use drugs acting through different mechanisms (i.e. an aqueous humor production inhibitor and a drug that increases the uveoscleral outflow).

All drugs have side-effects, although they may vary in frequency and severity. To decrease systemic absorption of the drug and increase ocular penetration, patients should be encouraged to do punctal occlusion. This maneuver is accomplished by applying digital pressure against the nose where the two lids come together for 2–3 minutes with the eyelids gently closed. When done correctly, punctal occlusion reduces drainage onto the nasal mucosa and systemic absorption (Figure 11.1) while prolonging drug-corneal contact time and intraocular absorption. (Further guidelines are described in Chapter 15.)

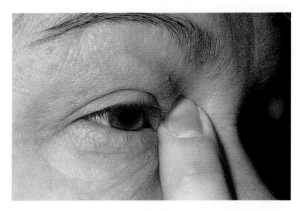

Figure 11.1 Punctal nasolacrimal occlusion. If digital pressure is placed over the area of the puncta and nasolacrimal duct after instilling a topical medication, passage of non-absorbed medication down the duct and into the nose will be reduced, thus decreasing systemic absortion and the potential for systemic side-effects. This maneuver should be combined with simple eyelid closure for a period of 1 to 2 min, which decreases the movement of tears (and medication dissolved in them) towards the puncta.

Cholinergic agents

For more than 100 years, ophthalmologists have been using cholinergic drugs to treat glaucoma. This group of drugs, which mimic and amplify the parasympathetic nervous system, can be divided into two groups, based on the site of action. Drugs such as pilocarpine, acetylcholine hydrochloride and carbachol, act directly at the neuromuscular junction. Indirect-acting parasympathomimetics, such as demecarium bromide, echothiophate iodide, and diidopropyl fluorophosphate, also known as anticholinesterase agents, bind to acetylcholinesterase and prevent the breakdown of acetylcholine at the neuromuscular junction, resulting in a buildup of acetylcholine and stimulation of the parasympathetic nervous system.

Pilocarpine

Cholinergic stimulation of the ciliary muscle by pilocarpine results in traction on the scleral spur, altering the configuration of the trabecular meshwork and leading to enhanced outflow and reduced IOP. Pilocarpine is available at a wide range of concentrations, of which the 1%, 2%, and 4% solutions are most commonly used. The maximal IOP reduction occurs at 2 hours, with the magnitude and duration of the fall being dependent on the concentration. Although

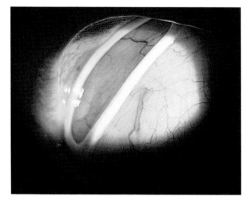

Figure 11.2 Ocusert system in the upper fornix. Ocusert is a semi-permeable membrane system, which slowly releases pilocarpine over 1 week when left in place in the conjunctival fornix. Reproduced with permission from Robin AL, Novack GD, Choplin NT. Medical therapy for glaucoma. In: Chopin NT, Lundy DC, eds. Atlas of Glaucoma. London; Martin Dunitz, 1998.

the duration of action varies between 6 and 8 hours and the standard regimen is four times daily, it is recommended that the frequency of administration should be titrated for each patient.

The Ocusert is a membrane-controlled delivery system with zero order pharmacokinetics. It is placed in the superior or inferior cul-de-sac (Figure 11.2) and delivers a constant rate of 20 micrograms per hour (Ocusert P-20), or 40 micrograms per hour (Ocusert P-40), which is roughly equivalent to 1–2% and 2–4% pilocarpine, respectively. The system delivers one-fifth of the amount of medicine required by drops for a similar IOP reduction. This makes it particularly useful in younger patients, who do not tolerate brisk variations in pupil diameter and ciliary spasm. The Ocusert is used every 5 to 7 days depending upon effect.

Pilocarpine can also be given in a high viscosity vehicle (Pilo HS Gel), designed to be used normally at bedtime. At this time, the side-effects induced by pilocarpine are less bothersome for the patient. 50 microliters of the gel contains 2 mg pilocarpine and is equivalent to a 50 microliter drop of 4% pilocarpine solution.

Carbachol, having both a direct and indirect action, is a more potent parasympathetic agent with a longer duration of action. It is usually given three times a day, but with punctal occlusion for 3 min after instillation, it can be used twice a day. Available commercially in 0.75%, 1.5%, and 3% solutions, it is primarily used when a patient develops an allergy to pilocarpine and requires a miotic agent. Because the 3% solution is far above the dose-response curve, this strength is rarely used.

Miotic drugs may cause a transitory conjunctival hyperemia due to vasodilation of conjunctival vessels. Miosis and ciliary spasm are the most common ocular side-effects, resulting in dim vision, myopia, and a typical brow ache which tends to disappear after the first week of treatment. Miotics are poorly tolerated by patients with cortical or subcapsular lens opacities. Ciliary muscle contraction also results in axial thickening of the lens, leading to shallowing of the anterior chamber and thereby allowing a phacomorphic closure of the anterior chamber angle in predisopsed eyes. Therefore, during chronic miotic therapy, periodic gonioscopy is vital to exclude miotic-induced angle closure.

Cholinergic-induced dilation of anterior segment vessels is associated with a breakdown in the blood–aqueous barrier and ciliary body congestion. The first explains why miotics should be avoided in situations where the blood–aqueous barrier is already compromised (i.e. uveitic glaucoma, neovascular glaucoma). The latter may augment the shallowing of the anterior chamber because the lens–iris diaphragm is pulled closer to the scleral spur by the contraction of the longitudinal muscle of the ciliary body. Contraction of the circular muscle of the ciliary body takes the tension off the zonules, allowing the lens to become more spherical and move more anteriorly, enhancing pupil block or aqueous misdirection in predisposed eyes.

Retinal detachment has been associated with cholinergic agents, especially in eyes with other risk factors such as myopia, aphakia, or lattice degeneration. It is thus recommended that a careful retinal examination should be done before the initiation of miotic therapy.

Excessive doses of pilocarpine may result in muscarinic poisoning, characterized by diarrhea, salivation, bradycardia, diaphoresis, nausea and vomiting. These signs and symptoms are more frequent when anticholinesterase agents are employed. However, in the latter situation, nicotinic poisoning may also develop, resulting in weakness, muscular twitching, cramps, pallor, tremor, and confusion.

Indirect-acting drugs

Anticholinesterase agents have been used in the treatment of glaucoma since the 1950s. They are generally more potent than pilocarpine, and are associated with more important side-effects. For this reason, they have not been used routinely in glaucoma treatment for the past 20 years. Phospholine iodide 0.06% is more potent than pilocarpine 4%. As with carbachol 3%, phospholine iodide at 0.25% is far above the dose-response curve and causes more inflammation without any additional effect, compared with the 0.06% solution in eyes with light irides and 0.125% in eyes with dark irides. Maximal IOP reduction occurs within 24 hours, lasting from several days to 2 weeks.

The ocular side-effects of indirect-acting cholinergic drugs are similar to those of pilocarpine, but in many cases more profound. Anticholinesterase agents promote an intense and prolonged miosis, which can be observed 30 minutes after instillation, and may lead to iris cysts. The cysts are more common in children and with the use of echothiophate and isoflurophate. They may cause visual distortion, but tend to resolve when therapy is discontinued. Cholinesterase inhibitors may also cause stenosis of the lacrimal punctum, resulting in epiphora.

Anticholinesterase agents have also been associated with anterior subcapsular cataracts. It is thought that inhibition of acetylcholinesterase in the lens capsule may increase lens hydration and upset the ionic balance and oxygen consumption, resulting in anterior subcapsular cataract.

Plasma cholinesterase causes the hydrolysis of several anesthetics, including procaine, tetracaine, and dibucaine. In addition, succinylcholine, a muscle relaxant commonly used to induce general anesthesia, is also inactivated by acetylcholinesterase. Glaucoma patients treated with indirect-acting miotics might experience prolonged apnea if succinylcholine is used during general anesthesia. For this reason, anticholinesterase agents should be discontinued 6 weeks before surgery.

Epinephrine and dipivefrin

The receptors that regulate sympathetic activity at various organs are known as α and β receptors. β receptors are classified as $\beta1$ or $\beta2$, and α receptors are subdivided as $\alpha1$ or $\alpha2$. Epinephrine (adrenaline) is a non-selective α and β-adrenergic agonist, which was first used as an antiglaucoma drug in the 1920s. The mechanism of action of epinephrine is not fully understood, although it is known that an improvement in conventional outflow, probably mediated by $\beta2$ adrenergic receptors, is its main effect. An epinephrine-mediated increase in uveoscleral outflow has also been described.

Epinephrine can reduce IOP by 10–30%, with the effect being greatest at 2–6 hours, and persisting for 12–24 hours after instillation, justifying a b.i.d. dosing schedule. Epinephrine is commercially available in three preparations with similar IOP lowering effects: hydrochloride, borate, and bitartrate at concentrations from 0.5–2%. Epinephrine is also available as the prodrug dipivefrin (dipivalyl-epinephrine hydrochloride), a compound which is more lipophilic, increasing corneal penetration and allowing the use of 0.1% concentration (Propine®). Dipivefrin is hydrolized to epinephrine in the cornea and has the same IOP lowering effects as epinephrine 1%. Its onset of action is 30 minutes, with the peak effect at 1 hour.

With the advent of new antiglaucoma drugs, the use of epinephrine and dipivefrin has become progressively less popular, mainly due to their ocular side-effects. Instillation of epinephrine leads to an immediate conjunctival vasoconstriction, followed by rebound vasodilation and conjunctival hyperemia. Common ocular side-effects include the development of allergy, characterized by follicular conjunctivitis, and blepharitis with or without periocular skin involvement.

165

patients with asthma or chronic obstructive pulmonary disease. Although betax-olol has been shown to be better tolerated than non-specific β blockers in patients with pulmonary disease, it should not be used in patients on medication for asthma. Betaxolol apparently has less important CNS side-effects than timolol, and does not appear to reduce exercise-induced heart rate.

Alpha-agonists

Clonidine

Clonidine was the first relatively selective α2 agonist to be used in the treatment of glaucoma. However, due to its lipophilic profile, which allows a rapid passage through the blood–brain barrier, systemic side-effects such as orthostatic hypotension and a significant reduction in resting blood pressure are frequently observed. These effects are thought to be a consequence of the stimulation of the presynaptic α2 receptors in the vasomotor centers of the brain, resulting in inhibition of sympathetic activity and peripheral vasodilation.

Clonidine 0.25% and 0.5% effectively reduce IOP, but the significant blood pressure decrease observed as early as 1 week after the start of therapy has limited its use in ophthalmology, and has stimulated the development of different α2 agonists with less important systemic side-effects. Nevertheless, topical clonidine hydrochloride 0.125%, 0.25%, and 0.5% (prescribed three times daily) is still available in some European countries.

Apraclonidine

Apraclonidine hydrochloride (Iopidine®) is an amino derivative of clonidine and is a relatively selective α2 agonist with minimal adverse systemic cardiovascular effects. Apraclonidine is less lipophilic than clonidine, which decreases its penetration across the blood-brain barrier and causes fewer CNS-mediated side effects.

Apraclonidine lowers IOP by reducing aqueous humor production by up to 35%, without changing aqueous outflow. The mechanisms involved in the reduction of aqueous humor production are not completely understood, although part of its effect may be secondary to an α1-mediated vasoconstriction of the ciliary body. Apraclonidine 1% produces a rapid drop in IOP within 1 hour of instillation, leading to a 30–40% IOP reduction after 3–5 hours. Apraclonidine is commercially available in concentrations of 0.5% for chronic use and 1% for prevention of IOP spikes after laser procedures (posterior capsulotomy, trabeculoplasty, iridotomy). When used to prevent IOP spikes, apraclonidine 1% should

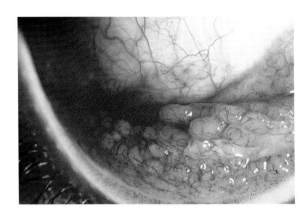

Figure 11.3
Allergic follicular
reaction of the
inferior tarsal
conjunctiva after
treatment with
topical brimonidine.

be instilled 1 hour before and immediately after the procedure. In a double-masked, randomized study, apraclonidine 1% reduced the incidence of IOP spikes greater than 10 mmHg from 17.6% in the placebo-treated group to 0% in eyes undergoing argon laser trabeculoplasty (ALT).

When used chronically, apraclonidine may be instilled twice daily or three times daily. In a 90-day study comparing timolol 0.5% b.i.d., apraclonidine 0.25% t.i.d., and apraclonidine 0.5% t.i.d., the IOP lowering effect was not significantly different between the groups. However, 36% of the patients receiving apraclonidine 0.5% were withdrawn from the study due to an allergic-like reaction characterized by discomfort, hyperemia, itching, tearing, foreign body sensation, follicles, and edema of the lids and conjunctiva (Figure 11.3). This allergic reaction typically starts weeks to months after the initiation of therapy, and normally disappears 3–5 days after medication is stopped. These side-effects may occur in up to 50% of patients, and limit the use of apraclonidine as primary therapy. This led the FDA to approve apraclonidine 0.5% for topical administration as an additive drug for patients receiving maximum-tolerated medical therapy. Its use has been greatly reduced by the introduction of newer $\alpha 2$ agonists.

Some authors have suggested that tachyphylaxis develops after the chronic use of apraclonidine. Robin and colleagues described a diminished IOP decrease over time, but could not determine whether this finding was indicative of tachyphylaxis or disease progression. Although apraclonidine is classed as an $\alpha 2$ agonist, it also stimulates $\alpha 1$ receptors, leading to conjunctival blanching, midryasis, and lid retraction—effects which tend to be subtle and transitory. The most common systemic side-effect of apraclonidine is dry mouth or dry nose, secondary to vasoconstriction of the nasal and oral mucosa, which affects about 5–20% of patients. Apraclonidine has minimal cardiovascular side-effects, although 5–10% of the patients may report fatigue.

Brimonidine

Brimonidine is a less lipophilic analog of clonidine, which provides clinically significant lowering of IOP. Brimonidine is a potent α-adrenoceptor agonist that is 1000-fold more selective for $\alpha2$ than the $\alpha1$ adrenoceptor, 7–12-fold more $\alpha2$-selective than clonidine and 23–32-fold more $\alpha2$-selective than apracloni-dine.

Brimonidine tartrate 0.2% (Alphagan®) promotes a mean IOP reduction of 20–25% at peak. It may be instilled two or three times daily, the latter regimen resulting in an additional IOP reduction in the afternoon. Combined data from two multicenter studies comparing brimonidine 0.2% b.i.d. with timolol 0.5% b.i.d. showed no significant differences between the groups at peak (2 hours after instillation), except for weeks 1 and 2 and month 3, when brimonidine resulted in lower mean IOPs. However, at trough (12 hours after instillation), timolol promoted significantly lower IOPs.

Brimonidine 0.5% was effective in preventing post-ALT IOP spikes in two multicenter studies. Only 1–2% of patients receiving brimonidine before and immediately after ALT had IOP spikes within the first 3 postoperative hours, compared with 23% of those on placebo.

Since brimonidine is a highly selective $\alpha2$ agonist, side-effects associated with $\alpha1$ adrenoceptor stimulation are less common. Furthermore, the incidence of ocular allergy observed with brimonidine (10–15%) is lower than that induced by apraclonidine (36%), probably because the first is oxidatively stable.

Brimonidine 0.2% is not associated with significant changes in systolic blood pressure or heart rate, although diastolic blood pressure reduction has been described. Patients receiving brimonidine may complain of dry mouth (30%), fatigue and drowsiness (16%), and headache (18%).

Carbonic anhydrase inhibitors

Systemic

Oral carbonic anhydrase inhibitors (CAIs) have been in clinical use for over 40 years, after the observation that acetazolamide lowered the IOP of glaucoma patients. This group of drugs acts by inhibiting the isoenzime CAI-II in the ciliary body epithelia, decreasing the rate of appearance of newly formed bicarbonate and sodium in the posterior chamber, and reducing the production of aqueous humor without changing the outflow facility.

Oral CAIs such as acetazolamide and methazolamide are very effective ocular hypotensive agents. The recommended oral dosage of acetazolamide (Diamox®) for chronic therapy in adults is 125 or 250 mg tablets every 6 hours, or 500 mg sustained release capsules every 12 hours. The peak effect with tablets occurs at

2 hours and lasts up to 6 hours. The peak effect with capsules occurs at 8 hours and lasts up to 12 hours. Methazolamide is administered with 25 mg or 50 mg tablets 2 to 4 times daily.

The extraocular inhibition of the enzyme results in metabolic acidosis and a myriad of side-effects, which include fatigue, depression, decreased sexual libido, metallic taste to foods, gastritis, paresthesias, weight loss, renal calculi, and nocturia. Rare but life-threatening complications include erythema multiforme and aplastic anemia. As a consequence of this, about 50% of patients receiving oral CAIs are unable to continue therapy. With the development of topical CAIs (see below) and other glaucoma drugs, the use of oral CAIs has become increasingly less popular.

Dorzolamide

A natural approach to decreasing the systemic side-effects associated with oral CAIs was the development of a topical CAI. In 1995, dorzolamide became the first topical CAI to be available clinically for the treatment of glaucoma.

Dorzolamide 2% (Trusopt®) produces its peak effect 2 hours after instillation (25% IOP reduction), whereas at trough, the IOP lowering effect is slightly reduced to 19%.

The ocular hypotensive effect of dorzolamide has been compared with timolol 0.5% and betaxolol 0.5% b.i.d. At 1 year, there were no significant differences at peak (23%, 25%, and 21% IOP reduction for dorzolamide, timolol, and betaxolol, respectively). At trough (8 hours post-dosing), the corresponding IOP reductions were 17%, 20%, and 15%, with the effect of timolol being significantly greater than dorzolamide and betaxolol. As adjunctive therapy, dorzolamide 2% is effective when associated with timolol, latanoprost, and patients receiving maximal medical therapy.

Patients given dorzolamide experience ocular burning and stinging, and may develop follicular conjunctivitis and eyelid edema. As expected, systemic side-effects after the use of dorzolamide are rare, the most common being a transient bitter taste reported by 27% of patients.

Brinzolamide

Brinzolamide is another topical CAI commercially available as a 1% suspension (Azopt®). A double-masked, prospective, parallel study compared brinzolamide 1% twice or three times daily, dorzolamide 2% three times daily, and timolol 0.5% twice daily, in 572 patients with ocular hypertension or glaucoma. At the end of the 3-month follow-up, the mean IOP reduction observed with dorzolamide and brinzolamide were similar both at peak (21–22% with brinzolamide, 23% with dorzolamide) and trough (17–19% with brinzolamide and 18% with dorzolamide).

171

Brinzolamide has a pH of about 7.5, which is less acidic than the dorzolamide 2% solution (pH 4.5). The difference in pH leads to a lower incidence of ocular burning and stinging when brinzolamide is used (3% vs 16% for dorzolamide). However, being a suspension, brinzolamide is associated with a higher rate of blurred vision (3.6% vs 0.6% with dorzolamide).

Prostaglandin-related drugs

Prostaglandin-related drugs have been investigated for decades because of their possible IOP lowering effect. Different prostanoids may induce a variety of side-effects in the human eye, ranging from mild conjunctival hyperemia to an initial ocular hypertensive response. In 1985, the first study to investigate the use of prostanoids in human volunteers tested a high dose (200 µg) of the tromethamine salt of PGF2α. Unfavorable side-effects such as ocular pain, conjunctival hyperemia, and headache discouraged its use in chronic therapy. It became clear that the elimination of these side-effects would require the chemical modification of the PGF2α moiety. Initially, the investigation of pulmonary PG metabolites resulted in the development of isopropyl unoprostone. Later, the 17-phenyl substituted PGF2α analogues (PhXA34 and latanoprost) were found to provide the most acceptable separation between ocular hypotensive efficacy and ocular side-effects.

Latanoprost

Latanoprost is a lipophilic, esterified prodrug, which is inactive until it undergoes enzymatic hydrolysis in the cornea, becoming the biologically active acid of latanoprost. The mechanism of action of latanoprost is different from the other drugs previously used to treat primary open angle glaucoma (POAG), since it has no effect on aqueous humor production or the conventional outflow. Latanoprost lowers IOP by increasing uveoscleral outflow, which has been demonstrated in animal eyes by tracer techniques, and in human eyes using indirect assessment of uveoscleral outflow.

Dose finding studies suggested that low concentrations were close to the top dose-response curve for latanoprost. Dose regimen studies revealed that once-daily administration of latanoprost 0.005% (Xalatan®) was at least as effective as twice-daily administration, with mean IOP reductions of 36% and 28%, respectively.

Several phase III clinical trials showed that latanoprost 0.005% instilled once daily is highly effective in reducing IOP in patients with POAG and OH, and that latanoprost is at least as effective as timolol maleate 0.5% (Table 11.1).

Table 11.1

	Baseline IOP (mmHg)	IOP Reduction at 6 months (mmHg)) [%]
Scandinavia		
Latanoprost (n = 183)	25.1 ± 3.5	8.0 ± 3.1 [32]*
Timolol (n = 84)	24.6 ± 3.1	6.4 ± 3.1 [26]
UK		
Latanoprost (n = 149)	25.2 ± 3.4	8.5 ± 2.8 [34]
Timolol (n = 145)	25.4 ± 3.6	8.4 ± 3.5 [33]
USA		
Latanoprost (n = 128)	24.4 ± 3.2	6.7 ± 3.4 [28]*
Timolol (n = 140)	24.1 ± 3.6	4.9 ± 2.9 [20]
Japan		
Latanoprost (n = 80)	23.1 ± 1.9	6.2 ± 2.7 [27]*
Timolol (n = 83)	23.1 ± 1.7	4.4 ± 2.3 [19]

Latanoprost has an additional IOP lowering effect when associated with other anti-glaucoma medications such as betablockers, carbonic anhydrase inhibitors, and dipivefrin. Although pilocarpine strongly decreases uveoscleral outflow, an additive effect is frequently observed when latanoprost is combined with pilocarpine.

The most common ocular symptoms after the use of latanoprost include foreign body sensation (13.3%), stinging (9.3%), and itching and burning (7.5%). In addition, punctate keratitis is seen in about 10% of latanoprost-treated eyes, which may be secondary to a higher concentration (0.02%) of benzalkonium chloride, used as a preservative. Latanoprost causes an increase in iridial pigmentation in some patients, particularly those with green or blue irides with a brownish peri-pupillary halo and those with light brown irides (Figure 11.4A). This complication affects 12% of patients (including all ranges of iris colors). However, if the predisposed irides are analysed separately, the probability of developing iris color change increases to 20% in blue-brown eyes, and 50% in green-brown or yellow-brown eyes after 1 year. The iris color change is secondary to an increased melanogenesis, with more melanin being produced by the melanocytes in the iris stroma. Although no further darkening of the iris has been observed following the discontinuation of the drug, the change is apparently permanent. Iris nevi or freckles may not be affected by latanoprost.

Other local side-effects include thickening and increase in the number of eyelashes (Figure 11.4B), increased pigmentation of periorbital skin, and transitory conjunctival hyperemia. Recently, some reports of anterior uveitis and cystoid macular edema in eyes with a previous history of uveitis or ocular surgery were attributed to latanoprost. Although there is no latanoprost-induced change in the blood–aqueous and blood–retinal barrier in normal eyes, a recent

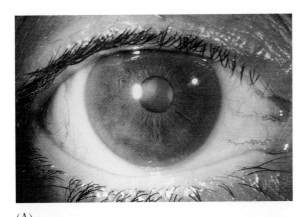

(A)

Figure 11.4A and 11.4B Latanoprost-induced iris hyperpigmentation (A-top and A-bottom)

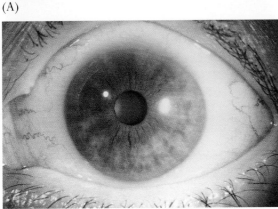

(A)

study showed that both barriers may be affected by latanoprost in eyes undergoing cataract surgery. These reports suggest that latanoprost needs to be used with caution in eyes where the blood–aqueous barrier is already compromised, especially in aphakic/pseudophakic eyes (i.e. uveitic glaucoma, neovascular glaucoma).

Another potential complication associated with latanoprost use is the recurrence of herpetic keratitis. Wand and colleages first described three cases in which herpes simplex keratitis developed after the start of latanoprost therapy. Subsequently, an experimental study in rabbits confirmed that latanoprost may worsen acute herpetic keratitis in the rabbit eye and increase the risk of recurrence in latently infected animals.

The systemic side-effects attributed to latanoprost are rare. In dose-tolerance studies, latanoprost has been administered intravenously to healthy volunteers at a dosage of 3 g/kg. Despite plasma concentrations 200 times greater than those obtained after instillation, no adverse reactions were noted. Systemic side-effects

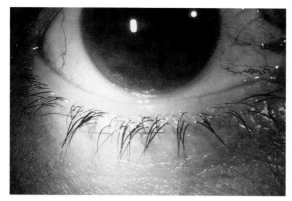

and eyelashes growth
(B-top, B-bottom)
compared with the
fellow eye after
unilateral treatment.

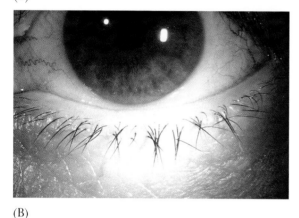

(B)

associated with prostaglandins (i.e. uterine contraction) are not observed, since the plasma levels reached after the instillation of such a small concentration are very low. However, it should not be used in pregnant women.

Isopropyl unoprostone

Isopropyl unoprostone (Rescula®) is a derivative of a prostaglandin metabolite that decreases IOP. It has been used in Japan since 1994. Unoprostone, which is classified as a docosanoid, contains 22 carbon atoms and a keto group at C-15, whereas latanoprost and primary prostaglandins are classified as eicosanoids with 20 carbon atoms and a keto group at C-15. Unoprostone is hydrolysed during its passage through the cornea by esterases, resulting in a free carboxylic acid, which is the pharmacologically active substance. Unoprostone and its free acid were shown to have no binding affinity to human prostanoid receptors (FD, DP, IP, TP, EP1, EP2, Table 11.1).

175

There is not enough experimental evidence to define conclusively the way in which unoprostone exerts its IOP lowering effect. Although no changes have been shown in aqueous humor production, there is still some controversy about unoprostone's effect on aqueous outflow. Some authors have reported an increase in aqueous outflow via the conventional (trabecular) pathway, whereas others have speculated that unoprostone might increase outflow via the uveoscleral or via both uveoscleral and conventional pathways.

A double-masked study in Japan, including 158 glaucoma and ocular hypertension patients and comparing 0.12% unoprostone instilled twice daily to timolol maleate 0.5% twice daily for 12 weeks, showed that both resulted in a significant IOP reduction (5.2 mmHg and 5.4 mmHg, respectively), and that unoprostone was at least as effective as timolol maleate. However, multicenter clinical trials in the USA and Europe showed that unoprostone 0.15% instilled twice daily was less effective than timolol 0.5%, but as effective as betaxolol 0.5%.

Yamamoto and colleagues showed that unoprostone 0.12% b.i.d and pilocarpine 1% q.i.d had similar IOP lowering effects, and that the addition of pilocarpine to ongoing unoprostone therapy resulted in increased IOP reduction. Combined use of unoprostone 0.12% and timolol 0.5% was significantly more effective than the respective monotherapies in seven patients (14 eyes) with POAG or OH. Yoshida and colleagues should that pretreatment IOP and history of cataract surgery were significant prognostic factors in determining the responsiveness to unoprostone of POAG eyes previously treated with other drugs.

No major systemic side-effect has been reported among the estimated 250 000 patients treated with unoprostone since its introduction on the Japanese market in 1994. Animal experiments have not shown CNS, somatic nervous system, digestive tract, or cardiorespiratory disorders. Local side-effects associated with unoprostone include conjunctival hyperemia in 6%, itching and burning in 5%, superficial keratitis (1.2%), and corneal epithelial damage (1–10%). An experimental study in cynomolgus monkeys showed that increased iris pigmentation was not observed 3 months after the instillation of unoprostone, but occurred in 100% of the cases when latanoprost was used. In humans, there have been reports of iris pigmentation, one of them diagnosed 20 months after the start of unoprostone therapy. There have been some recent isolated reports of anterior uveitis, thickening and increase in number of eyelashes. Long-term, comparative studies are needed to assess whether the incidence of such side-effects is lower than that observed with latanoprost.

Bimatoprost and travaprost

Recently, two new prostaglandin derivatives were introduced to the market. Both of them are instilled once daily and seem to show similar hypotensive efficacy compared to latanoprost.

176

Fixed combination therapy

Fixed combination therapies may enhance compliance and the quality of life by decreasing the number of instillations per day, maintaining the hypotensive efficacy with fewer drops. In general, combinations have to fulfill some requirements. The efficacy of a fixed combination of drug A and drug B has to be greater than drug A or drug B alone. Although a complete additive effect is not required by the FDA, the ideal fixed combination would have the same effect of the concomitant use of drug A and drug B. Several fixed combinations have been developed, including timolol-pilocarpine, epinephrine-pilocarpine, and betaxolol-pilocarpine. A fixed combination of dorzolamide 2% and timolol (Cosopt®) 0.5% is now commercially available in several countries. An experimental study in rabbits has shown that the ocular penetration of one drug is not affected by the other, leading to similar concentrations of dorzolamide and timolol in the ciliary body of rabbits after the instillation of the fixed combination and of both drugs individually.

A 3-month, double-masked study including 335 patients compared the efficacy and safety of the fixed combination instilled twice daily with the individual components (timolol 0.5% b.i.d, and dorzolamide 2% t.i.d). At the end of the follow-up period, the mean IOP reduction at peak was 32.7%, 19.8%, and 22.6% for the fixed combination, dorzolamide 2%, and timolol 0.5%, respectively. The clinical efficacy of the fixed combination was similar to the concomitant administration of its two components in a double-masked study with 242 patients with glaucoma or ocular hypertension. After 3 months, the IOP reduction relative to the timolol 0.5% baseline was 14% at hour 0, 20% at hour 2, and 15% at hour 8, compared with 16%, 20%, and 17% with the concomitant therapy. This study also showed that the fixed combination maintained a consistent IOP reduction over 1 year.

Suggested reading

Alm A, Stjernschantz J, The Scandinavian Latanoprost Study Group. Effects on intraocular pressure and side effects of 0.005% latanoprost once daily, evening or morning. A comparison with timolol. *Ophthalmology* 1995;**102**:1743–52.

Azuma I, Masuda K, Kitazawa K. Double-masked, comparative study of UF-021 and timolol ophthalmic solutions in patients with primary open-angle glaucoma or ocular hypertension. *Jpn J Ophthalmol* 1993;**37**:514–25.

Azuma I, Masuda K, Kitazawa K. Late phase II clinical study of UF-021 ophthalmic solution in primary open angle glaucoma and ocular hypertension. *Nippon Ganka Gakkai Zasshi* 1992;**96**:1261–7.

Becker B. Decrease in intraocular pressure in man by a carbonic anhydrase inhibitor. Diamox. *Am J Ophthalmol* 1954;**37**:13–5.

Becker B, Gage T. Demecarium bromide and echothiophate iodide in chronic glaucoma. *Arch Ophthalmol* 1960;**63**:126–31.

Boyle JE, Ghosh K, Gieser DK et al. A randomized trial comparing the dorzolamide-timolol combination given twice daily to monotherapy with timolol and dorzolamide. *Ophthalmology* 1998;**105**:1945–51.

Butler P, Mannschreck M, Lin S et al. Clinical experience with the long-term use of 1% apraclonidine. Incidence of allergic reactions. *Arch Ophthalmol* 1995;**113**:293–6.

Drance SM, Nash PA. The dose response of human intraocular pressure to pilocarpine. *Can J Ophthalmol* 1971;**6**:9–13.

Drance SM, Ross RA. The ocular effects of epinephrine. *Surv Ophthalmol* 1970;**14**:330–5.

Fellman RL, Starita RJ. Ocular and systemic side effects of topical cholinergic and anticholinesterase drugs. In Sherwood MB, Spaeth GL. Complications of Glaucoma Therapy. Thorofare, NJ: Slack Incorporated, 1990; 5–18.

Kass MA, Mandell AI, Goldberg I et al. Dipivefrin and epinephrine treatment of elevated intraocular pressure. A comparative study. *Arch Ophthalmol* 1979;**97**:1865–6.

Katz LJ. Brimonidine tartrate 0.2% twice daily vs timolol 0.5% twice daily: 1-year results in glaucoma patients. *Am J Ophthalmol* 1999;**127**:20–6.

Michels RG, Maumenee E. Cystoid macular edema associated with topically applied epinephrine in aphakic eyes. *Am J Ophthalmol* 1975;**80**:379–88.

Miyake K, Ota I, Maekubo K et al. Latanoprost accelerates disruption of the blood aqueous barrier and the incidence of angiographic cystoid macular edema in early postoperative pseudophakias. *Arch Ophthalmol* 1999;**117**:34–40.

Novak GD. Ophthalmic beta-blockers since timolol. *Surv Ophthalmol* 1987;**31**:307–27.

Silver LH. The Brinzolamide Primary Therapy Study Group. Clinical efficacy and safety of brinzolamide, a new topical carbonic anhydrase inhibitor for primary open-angle glaucoma and ocular hypertension. *Am J Ophthalmol* 1998;**126**:400–8.

Stewart WC, Laibovitz R, Horwitz B et al. A 90-day study of the efficacy and side effects of 0.25% and 0.5% apraclonidine vs 0.5% timolol. *Arch Ophthalmol* 1996;**114**:938–42.

Strahlman E, Tipping R, Vogel R. The International Dorzolamide Study Group. A double-masked, randomized, 1-year study comparing dorzolamide, timolol, and betaxolol. *Arch Ophthalmol* 1995;**113**:1009–16.

Strohmaier K, Snyder E, DuBiner H et al. The efficacy and safety of the dorzolamide-timolol combination versus the concomitant administration of its components. *Ophthalmology* 1998;**105**:1936–44.

Taniguchi T, Haque MS, Sugiyama K. Ocular hypotensive mechanism of topical unoprostone isopropyl, a novel prostaglandin metabolite-related drug in rabbits. *J Ocul Pharmacol Ther* 1996;**12**:489–98.

The Levobunolol Study Group. Levobunolol: a beta-adrenoceptor antagonist effective in the long-term treatment of glaucoma. *Ophthalmology* 1985;**92**:1271–6.

Torris CB, Gleason ML, Camras CB et al. Effects of brimonidine on aqueous humor dynamics in human eyes. *Arch Ophthalmol* 1995;**113**:1514–17.

Torris CB, Tafoya ME, Camras CB et al. Effects of apraclonidine on aqueous humor dynamics in human eyes. *Ophthalmology* 1995;**102**:456–61.

Wand M, Gilbert CM, Liesegang G. Latanoprost and herpes simplex keratitis. *Am J Ophthalmol* 1999;**127**:602–4.

Watson P, Stjernschantz J, and the Latanoprost Study Group. A six-month, randomized, double masked study comparing latanoprost to timolol in open-angle glaucoma and ocular hypertension. *Ophthalmology* 1996;**103**:126–37.

Wistrand PJ, Stjernschantz J, Olsson K. The incidence and time-course of latanoprost-induced iridial pigmentation as a function of eye color. *Surv Ophthalmol* 1997;**41**(suppl 2):S129–38.

Zimmerman TJ, Kaufman HE. Timolol: A beta-adrenergic blocking agent for the treatment of glaucoma. *Arch Ophthalmol* 1977;**95**:601–4.

12. GLAUCOMA LASER PROCEDURES

Martha Motuz Leen

For the past three decades, lasers have enhanced the management of glaucomatous eyes. By modifying intraocular tissues while preserving surrounding ocular structures, the need for more invasive surgical procedures is often postponed or obviated. Lasers assist with intraocular pressure (IOP) control by either enhancing filtration (as with trabeculoplasty, iridotomy, iridoplasty, and sclerotomy) or by reducing aqueous production (as with cyclophotocoagulation).

Laser trabeculoplasty

Introduced in 1979, argon laser trabeculoplasty (ALT) is an effective means of lowering IOP by enhancing trabecular outflow in eyes with visible trabecular meshwork. Although the mechanism is only partially understood, it is widely believed that laser applications to trabecular meshwork create focal burns that contract the meshwork, increasing the size of adjacent intertrabecular spaces. The thermal effect may also stimulate phagocytosis, cellular proliferation or alter extracellular matrix. The argon laser is most commonly used for this procedure. A diode laser can be also used to do a trabeculoplasty.

Indications

ALT is most commonly performed in eyes with open angles that have inadequate control of IOP despite medical therapy. This includes eyes with ocular hypertension, primary open angle glaucoma, normal tension glaucoma and some types of secondary open angle glaucomas, particulary the pseudoexfoliative and pigmentary varieties. ALT in other types of open angle glaucomas, such as inflammatory, angle recession and juvenile varieties, is not recommended generally.

The typical succession of treatment consists of medication, then ALT, followed by filtration surgery. However, there is much flexibility in this sequence that can be tailored to an individual's needs. For instance, this procedure can be 1) offered earlier when cost, compliance, allergy or quality-of-life issues associated with medical therapy are problematic; 2) done in eyes with open angles that have had prior filtration surgery but not previous ALT; or 3) skipped entirely in preference for earlier surgery if a greater than 30% drop IOP is desired.

The Glaucoma Laser Trial, a multicenter randomized study, investigated the potential role of ALT as primary therapy compared with medical therapy in newly diagnosed primary open angle glaucoma. The study suggested that initial ALT may be at least as safe and effective as initial medical therapy after a median 7-year follow-up.

Technique

Preparation

Previous glaucoma medications are continued before treatment. The eye is anesthetized with a topical anesthetic. Apraclonidine is instilled 1 hour before and immediately after the laser treatment. Methylcellulose is dropped onto a 3-mirror Goldmann contact lens that is placed on the cornea. Visualization of the trabecular meshwork in a narrow angle can be optimized in one of three ways: 1) by asking the patient to look toward the treatment mirror; 2) by using the intermediate mirror of the Goldmann lens; or 3) by doing a laser iridotomy or laser peripheral iridoplasty first (see below). Compression with the Goldmann lens places pressure on the limbus, further narrowing the angle, and should be avoided. The aiming beam should be continuously refocused and round, with the beam placed in the center of the mirror to avoid an oval spot. The mirror is rotated to treat the desired quadrants.

Argon laser

The argon laser is set at a spot size of 50 microns, duration of 0.1 seconds and initial power of 400–800 mW. The trabecular meshwork is treated with laser energy delivered evenly spaced, totalling about 80–100 spots for a 360 degree treatment, or 40–50 spots for a 180 degree treatment. The burns are placed at the junction of the pigmented and non-pigmented trabecular meshwork, with power titrated continuously during the session to achieve a visible endpoint of mild blanching or small bubble formation (Figure 12.1). In general, meshwork with little pigment requires a higher power setting. Monochromatic green wavelength is preferable to blue-green wavelength to minimize risk of photoreceptor injury to the treating surgeon.

Postoperative management

The IOP is rechecked within the first 1–3 hours, and treated if a significant increase occurs. Preoperative glaucoma medications are continued. A topical corticosteroid drop is instilled 4 times a day for 7 days to minimize inflammation. The eye is re-examined 1 week later.

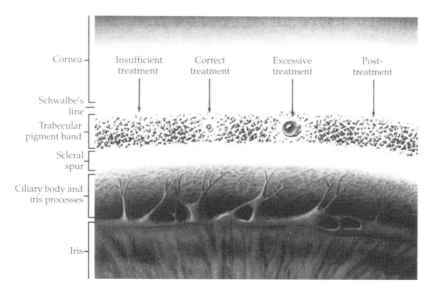

Figure 12.1 Laser trabeculoplasty. Formation of a small bubble at the junction of the pigmented and non-pigmented trabecular meshwork is the optimal response to argon laser treatment. *Reproduced with permission from: Schwartz AL, Whitten MF, Bleiman B, Martin D. Argon Laser trabecular surgery in uncontrolled phakic open angle glaucoma. Ophthalmology 1981;88:203–12.*

Complications

IOP increase can occur immediately after ALT. Although these spikes are usually transient, they can lead to visual field loss in eyes with advanced glaucomatous cupping. This risk is minimized with routine instillation of apraclonidine 0.5–1% before and after the procedure. Alternatively, brimonidine 0.5% can be administered in one dose either before or after the procedure. Risk factors for IOP increase include posterior laser applications, high power settings, and heavy trabecular pigmentation. Without apraclonidine use, the risk is higher with 360 degree treatment than with 180 degree treatment. However, with apraclonidine use, the risk is similar. Routinely doing two separate treatments should be weighed against the risk of exposing the eye to IOP spikes on two separate occasions.

A low grade anterior uveitis is expected and self-limiting. This is usually adequately controlled with postoperative instillation of topical steroid medication. In an eye with a propensity for inflammation, more aggressive topical steroid treatment would be indicated. A topical non-steroidal drop may be used as an alternative in eyes prone to steroid-induced IOP increases.

The contact lens used during treatment can cause corneal irritation and erosion, which usually responds to lubrication and resolves in 24 hours. Peripheral anterior synechaie after laser treatment are usually small, evenly spaced, with a peaked appearance. They are more common with posterior burn placement, higher power, narrow angles and dark irides.

Although the argon laser has a coagulative effect, a hyphema can occur infrequently when a prominent peripheral iris vessel is present, especially under anticoagulative medication. Rarely, pupil size may enlarge from a sector sphincter palsy at the pupillary margin.

Prognosis

The IOP response is best judged 6–8 weeks after treatment. The 1-year success rate of ALT is about 67–80%. The rate generally diminishes by 6–10% per year with success rates of 35–50% at 5 years and 5–30% at 10 years. The success of re-treatment is less than 50%, and is generally reserved for those who are not surgical candidates, or who have shown a good initial response to the first treatment.

The degree of trabecular pigmentation may correlate with better success. Pseudoexfoliative and pigmentary glaucomas, which have more angle pigmentation, tend to have better short-term success rates than primary open glaucoma, although the long-term effect degrades more rapidly. With the exception of pigmentary glaucoma, the success rate is lower in eyes less than 40 years old. The response rate is also lower in uveitic glaucoma and angle recession glaucoma. A good response can generally be expected if success was achieved in the contralateral eye.

Laser iridotomy

First introduced as an alternative to surgical iridectomy in 1956, laser iridotomy is done to relieve the pressure gradient between the anterior and posterior chambers of the eye. In classic 'pupillary block', the iris bows anteriorly due to higher aqueous pressure posterior to the iris, causing apposition of the iris against the trabecular meshwork. This may interfere with trabecular outflow, as seen with acute angle closure glaucoma. A small hole in the iris allows the pressure gradient between the anterior and posterior chambers to equalize, resulting in flattening of the iris curvature with opening of the angle (Figure 12.2). Laser iridotomy is usually done with the Nd:YAG laser by photodisruption, but can also be done with an argon laser in patients with bleeding tendencies via a thermal effect.

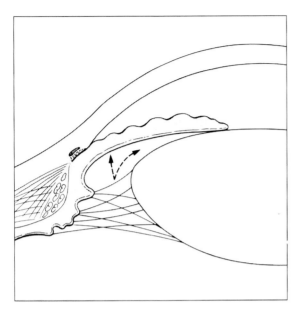

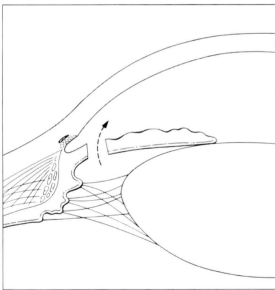

Figure 12.2 Laser iridotomy. Pupillary block occurs when there is contact between the iris and the lens, causing peripheral iris to bow forward and to block the trabecular meshwork (Above). A patent iridotomy allows the pressure gradient across the iris to equalize, resulting in a flattening of the iris bow and unblocking of the trabecular meshwork (Below). *Reproduced with permission from: Skuta GL. The angle closure glaucomas. In: Kaufman PL, Mittag TW (assoc. eds). Volume 7 Glaucoma. In: Podos SM, Yanoff M (eds). Textbook of Ophthalmology. Philadelphia: Mosby-Year Book, 1994;8.8–8.13.*

Indications

Laser iridotomy is most often performed in eyes that have appositionally occluded or occludable angles due to a classic pupillary block mechanism. This includes eyes with acute angle closure, history of acute angle closure in the fellow eye, subacute angle closure, intermittent angle closure, or occludable angles judged gonioscopically to be at risk of angle closure. These subsets of narrow angles may be primary in nature or have a secondary mechanism, such as with pupillary block due to pupillary synechiae from prior episodes of inflammation. Laser iridotomy is also indicated in eyes with suspected plateau iris, aqueous misdirection and phacomorphic narrowing to eliminate a pupillary block component before making the correct diagnosis. In cases in which corneal edema is severe or there is lack of cooperation from the patient, a surgical iridectomy may be the better option.

Technique

Preparation

Pilocarpine 1–2% is instilled before treatment to induce miosis, thinning the iris stroma. The eye is anesthetized with a topical anesthetic. Topical glycerin can be instilled if the view is hazy due to corneal edema. An apraclonidine drop is given 1 hour before and immediately after the procedure. If the eye is in an active episode of angle closure, appropriate medical therapy is instituted for IOP control. Methylcellulose is dropped onto an iridotomy lens that consists of a small planoconvex lens located on the peripheral portion of a contact lens. This lens is placed on the cornea and allows for enhanced magnification and focus, which is turn allows for more efficient delivery of laser energy.

Before treatment, the patient is asked to look down and the iris is visualized through the contact lens. An iris location is chosen in the superior position under the upper lid and preferably at the base of a crypt where the iris stroma is expected to be thin. To minimize the risk of lens damage, treatment should be as peripheral as possible. However, if a prominent corneal arcus is present, the treatment should be more central to minimize the risk of a corneal burn.

Nd:YAG laser

The laser is in the pulsed mode, with energy initially set at 4–6 mJ with 1–3 bursts per pulse. The spot size is constant within the laser unit. Since shock waves tend to be transmitted anteriorly, the aiming beam is focused within the iris stroma. As the treatment approaches the anterior lens capsule, the laser energy can be reduced to chip away the remaining stroma and minimize anterior capsular trauma. Once the iris pigment epithelium is penetrated in classic pupillary block, a visible burst of pigment with anterior aqueous flow is seen, with posterior movement and flattening of peripheral iris. The base of the iris pigment epithelium should be treated to allow an adequate size opening of 100–200 microns. Transillumination alone is not a reliable indicator of patency. The anterior lens capsule should be visualized through the iridotomy.

Argon laser

Alternatively, the argon laser can be used in patients with a tendency to bleeding, to pretreat the iridotomy location before using the Nd:YAG laser with lower energy settings, or to completely penetrate the iris. Pretreatment usually consists of a small ring of overlapping burns of 200 microns each with a pulse duration of 0.2–0.5 seconds, and a power intensity that will cause obvious constriction but not charring of the iris stroma. This pretreatment stretches the iris at the middle of the ring of burns and coagulates the blood vessels serving this area. Penetrating the iris with the argon laser is more difficult than with the Nd:YAG because the argon laser spot size is larger, with lower power density than the Nd:YAG. However, as the argon laser penetrates it also coagulates, minimizing the risk of bleeding from iris stromal vessels. The laser is set at a spot size of 50 microns, a duration of 0.01–0.02 seconds, and a power of 600–1200 mW. Since the argon laser produces a variable reaction depending upon the degree of pigmentation, the energy is adjusted according to response.

Postoperative management

The IOP is rechecked within the first 1–3 hours, and treated if a significant increase occurs. A topical corticosteroid drop is instilled 4 times a day for 3–7 days to minimize inflammation. Medical treatment for IOP control for an acute angle closure attack is instituted as needed. The eye is re-examined in one week, or sooner if the IOP is not stablized.

Complications

A transient rise of IOP immediately after the procedure may result from an excessive load of pigment, blood, or inflammatory debris on the trabecular meshwork. This risk is reduced with instillation of apraclonidine before and after the procedure.

A low grade anterior uveitis is expected. This is usually adequately controlled with postoperative instillation of topical steroid medication. The contact lens used during treatment can cause corneal irritation and abrasion, which usually respond to lubrication and resolve in 24 hours. Corneal endothelial damage can occur with a very shallow anterior chamber or with the presence of a corneal arcus. This may be associated with focal corneal edema that is usually transient.

Bleeding with hyphema formation is more common with the Nd:YAG laser. Once bleeding occurs, visualization of the iridotomy site can be compromised during treatment. Firm pressure can be placed on the eye with the contact lens until the bleeding has stopped. Argon laser pretreatment, which coagulates vessels, can minimize bleeding in those eyes judged to be at higher risk.

187

Functional iridotomy failure can occur if the iridotomy is too small, particularly < 50 microns, allowing a residual pressure gradient that does not adequately relieve pupillary block. Also, an iridotomy may appear to be of adequate size during treatment due to a burst of anterior aqueous flow and the stretching effect of a miotic pupil, but may decrease in size as the fluid flow slows and the pupil recovers its normal size. In such cases, the iridotomy can be enlarged with the laser. Late failure with closure of the hole is uncommon and can be seen as a result of proliferation of iris pigment epithelium, synechial closure, or membrane growth.

Macular damage is rare after iridotomy with the argon laser, but is at higher risk of occurring when a patent iridotomy is enlarged. The risk can be minimized by treating the superonasal quadrant of the iris, which would direct the laser beam away from the macula. The risk of anterior lens capsular rupture is greater with the YAG laser. This can result in focal opacities just beneath the anterior capsule, but does not appear to hasten the progression of cataract at a rate greater than that in the general population. Posterior synechiae at the pupillary margin can occur in eyes with excessive anterior chamber inflammation, especially with postoperative pilocarpine use. Glare and diplopia can occur if the iridectomy is not completely covered by the upper lid. Aqueous misdirection associated with miotic use is rare.

Prognosis

The success of an iridotomy is verified by establishing patency and confirming an anatomical widening of the angle by gonioscopy. The long-term efficacy of laser iridotomy is well documented and the iridotomy is expected to remain patent. Exceptions may include eyes with neovascular or uveitic glaucoma due to synechiae formation and membrane growth that can obscure an iridotomy. An angle that is initially open can become progressively narrower over time, despite a patent iridotomy, due to an increasing phacomorphic component associated with cataract progression.

In cases of angle closure attack, the IOP generally decreases immediately unless there is permanent damage to the trabecular meshwork from long-standing apposition. In others, the IOP is expected to remain unchanged, although future increases in IOP from angle closure are prevented. Additional medication or surgery is needed in 64% of eyes with acute angle closure, despite the presence of a patent iridotomy.

Laser peripheral iridoplasty

Laser peripheral iridoplasty was introduced in 1979 as a method for opening angles that remain appositionally closed despite the presence of a patent iridotomy. In

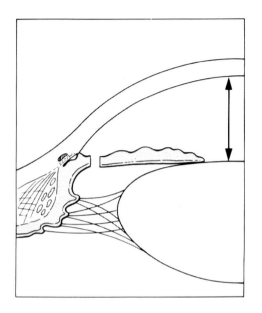

Figure 12.3 Plateau iris. The peripheral iris roll may continue to occlude the trabecular meshwork in the presence of a patent iridotomy. *Reproduced with permission from: Skuta GL. The angle closure glaucomas. In: Kaufman PL, Mittag TW (assoc. eds). Volume 7 Glaucoma. In: Podos SM, Yanoff M (eds). Textbook of Ophthalmology. Philadelphia: Mosby-Year Book, 1994, 8.15.*

these cases, mechanisms other than pupillary block are responsible for the narrow angle. The mechanism usually involves a peripheral iris that is pushed anteriorly due to ciliary body anatomy or lens position (Figure 12.3). A laser iridoplasty contracts iris stroma in the far periphery via low-power, large laser burns of long duration, flattening the peripheral iris convexity and alleviating the appositionally closed angle. This procedure is done with an argon laser.

Indications

In an angle that remains appositionally closed or occludable after a laser irido-tomy, a laser iridoplasty can open the residual angle closure. This situation can occur with plateau iris, in which the peripheral iris configuration is abnormally steep due to congenitally anterior positioning of the ciliary processes. Residual angle closure can also be related to angle crowding from an abnormally large or mobile lens as with lens intumescence or dislocation, or an abnormally small anterior segment, as with nanophthalmos. Anterior ciliary body rotation, result-ing from choroidal edema after scleral buckle or panretinal photocoagulation, can also crowd the angle. In these cases, laser iridoplasty may help open the angle by flattening the peripheral iris. Laser iridoplasty may also be useful before laser trabeculoplasty in an eye with a narrow angle, to better visualize the trabec-ular meshwork for treatment. Laser iridoplasty is not an appropriate treatment for peripheral anterior synechiae, flat anterior chamber, or anterior ciliary body rotation resulting from aqueous misdirection or choroidal detachment.

189

Technique

Preparation

Pilocarpine 1–2% is instilled before treatment, to induce miosis and to pull the iris away from the insertion. The eye is anesthetized with a topical anesthetic. Apraclonidine is given 1 hour before and immediately after the procedure. Methylcellulose is dropped onto a contact lens that consists of a small plano convex lens located on the peripheral portion of the lens. The lens is placed onto the eye.

Argon laser

The laser is set at a duration of 0.5 seconds, a spot size of 500 microns, and a power of 200–400 mW. The aiming beam is focused through the contact lens, onto the iris, as peripheral as possible. 20–24 laser burns are created evenly over 360 degrees (Figure 12.4). Lighter irides generally require more power than darker irides. The laser footpedal should be engaged for the entire 0.5 second duration. If bubble formation is seen, the power should be reduced. Focal iris contraction is visible during each treatment.

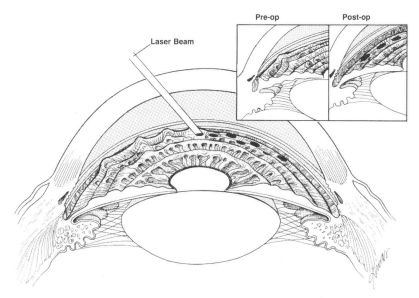

Figure 12.4 Laser peripheral iridoplasty. The laser treats peripheral iris, causing contraction and adjacent flattening of the peripheral iris roll.
Reproduced with permission from: Lindquist TD. Laser trabeculoplasty and iridoplasty. Lindquist TD, Lindstrom RL (eds). Ophthalmic Surgery. Chicago: Mosby-Year Book Medical Publishers, 5th edn, 1996:Section III-F-3.

Postoperative management

The IOP is rechecked within the first 1–3 hours, and treated if an increase occurs. A topical corticosteroid drop is instilled 4 times a day for 3–7 days to minimize inflammation. The eye is re-examined one week later.

Complications

As with laser iridotomy, there is risk of transient IOP increase, corneal irritation, corneal abrasion, corneal endothelial damage and anterior uveitis. Bleeding, however, is uncommon owing to the coagulative effects of the argon laser and lower power density.

Prognosis

IOP reduction after laser iridoplasty occurs in 63% of eyes treated for angle closure glaucoma unrelieved by a patent iridotomy. Anatomic success is verified gonioscopically. Burns that are mid-peripheral are more often associated with anatomical failure. If treatment is partially successful, or if the angle continues to narrow because of lens positioning, retreatment is done in a similar fashion, ideally between prior laser burns.

Transscleral laser cyclophotocoagulation

Laser cyclophotocoagulation can be done to lower IOP in selected cases of recalcitrant glaucoma by reducing aqueous production. Laser energy is delivered transsclerally to the ciliary body either through a contact mode with a fiberoptic probe, or through a non-contact method through a slit-lamp and contact lens. Aqueous formation is believed to be reduced directly through thermal destruction of ciliary body epithelium, and possibly indirectly from ciliary body vascular damage or uveitis. Transscleral cyclophotocoagulation is usually done with a Nd:YAG or diode laser, both of which depend upon absorption by pigment to achieve thermal effect, causing minimal damage to scleral integrity.

Indications

Transscleral laser cyclophotocoagulation is an option for lowering IOP in eyes with poor prognosis for filtration surgery, including those with neovascular glaucoma, uveitic glaucoma, congenital glaucomas, silicone oil-induced glaucoma (without pupillary block), or failed prior filtration surgery. This procedure can also be done in eyes with poor visual potential, severe pain or medical contraindications for filtration surgery. Since there is a significant risk of visual acuity loss associated with this procedure, it is used with caution in better-sighted eyes. The diode laser for the contact method and Nd:YAG laser for the non-contact method are commonly used for this procedure.

Techniques

Preparation

Previous glaucoma medications are continued before treatment. The eye is anesthetized with retrobulbar anesthesia. The eye can be transilluminated to confirm ciliary body location. The treatment is usually done for 270 degrees, avoiding the long posterior ciliary arteries at the 3 and 9 o'clock positions.

Contact method: diode laser

A wire speculum is placed. Different settings have been reported. We recommend the following protocol: For eyes with lightly colored irises, the diode laser is set at a duration of 3500 msec and a power of 1500 mW, each application being 5.25 J. For eyes with dark irides the duration is 4000 msec at 1.250 mW for a total of 5.0 J. 16–20 laser applications are delivered over 270 degrees using the fiberoptic G-probe placed with the anterior edge adjacent to the limbus (Figure 12.5). The probe is held parallel to the visual axis and firmly against the sclera. Thinner sclera generally requires lower energy settings, but areas of scleral atrophy should be avoided.

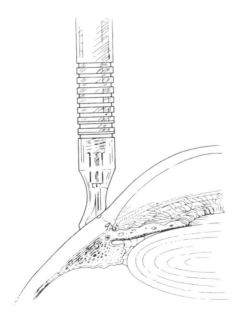

Figure 12.5

Contract transscleral cyclophotocoagulation. The G-probe is placed with the anterior edge adjacent to the limbus, delivering diode laser energy to the underlying ciliary body. *Permission to reprint pending from: Lewis RA. Transscleral laser cyclophotocoagulation. In: Mills RP, Weinreb RN (eds). Glaucoma Surgical Techniques. San Francisco: American Academy of Ophthalmology, 1998;165.*

If another treatment is required, 270 degrees can be treated again. This application is rotated 45° from the previous treatment so that half of the previously untouched quadrant is treated.

Non-contact method: Nd:YAG laser

The patient's head is positioned in the laser slit-lamp device. Methylcellulose is dropped onto a Shields Cyclophotocoagulation contact lens (Ocular Instruments, Bellevue, WA, USA) and placed firmly onto the eye in primary position, blanching conjunctival vessels around the limbus. The Nd:YAG Microrupter II laser (H.S Meridian, Inc, Mason, OH, USA) in the free-running mode is set at an energy of 4–8 J per pulse and maximal offset at 9 (separating laser focal point 3.6 mm beyond the aiming beam (Figure 12.6). 30–40 applications are delivered over 270–360 degrees, with the beam parallel to the visual axis and 1.5 mm posterior to the limbus. Transillumination allows better localization of the ciliary body and more accurate ablation. Etched lines on the contact lens are spaced at 1 mm intervals to help with beam location.

Postoperative management

Atropine 1% and steroid drops are instilled immediately after the procedure. Subtenons steroid injection can also be given to minimize inflammation. Topical

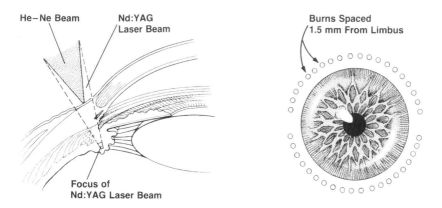

Figure 12.6 Non-contact transscleral cyclophotocoagulation. The aiming beam is directed 1.5 mm posterior to the limbus with the Nd:YAG laser beam offset posteriorly to reach the ciliary body (Left). Appearance of conjunctival blanching corresponding to laser treatments after completion of the procedure (Right) *Reproduced with permission from: Lindquist TD, Lindstrom RL (eds). Ophthalmic Surgery. Chicago: Mosby-Year Book Medical Publishers, 5th edn, 1996;Section III-D-6.*

glaucoma medications and sometimes osmotic agents may be required to prevent a postoperative intraocular pressure rise. If the postoperative pressure is satisfactory, the eye is patched for 6 hours over antibiotic ointment and examined the day after surgery. Topical steroid 4–8 times a day and atropine sulfate 1% twice daily are administered and readjusted as needed to control inflammation. Prior miotics and prostaglandins are discontinued. Other preoperative glaucoma medications can be continued, tapered or discontinued, depending upon the IOP response. The eye is re-examined in 1 week.

Complications

A mild to moderate uveitis, while expected, is usually transient, and is controlled with postoperative topical steroid therapy. Inflammation may be more prominent in eyes with a higher numbers of audible pops during the procedure. Occasionally a more severe inflammatory response with fibrin formation or hypopyon can occur, requiring more aggressive steroid therapy, especially in eyes with uveitic or neovascular glaucoma. Damage to the major arterial circle of the iris and long posterior ciliary vessels can cause hyphema or vitreous hemorrhage. Visual acuity loss occurs in 29–40% of eyes. Other complications include choroidal effusion, hypotony, conjunctival burns, postoperative IOP increase, corneal erosion, corneal graft failure, scleral thinning, aqueous misdirection, cystoid macular edema, pupillary distortion, cataract, and phthisis. Sympathetic ophthalmia has also been reported. In general, postoperative complications are less severe than with cyclocryotherapy.

Prognosis

Success rates with contact and non-contact methods are similar, and in the range of 52–84% and 45–73%, respectively. Both are at least as effective as cyclocryotherapy, with fewer complications. Repeat treatment is required in 45–49% of eyes. Improvement of visual acuity is rare. The success of this procedure is usually judged by IOP control, since it is often not a vision-saving procedure.

Laser sclerotomy

Laser sclerotomy is a means of creating full-thickness drainage fistulas with fewer complications than those reported with incisional full-thickness procedures (posterior lip sclerectomy, thermal sclerotomy) and with less tissue disruption than guarded filtration procedures (trabeculectomy). Laser energy can be delivered either internally (*ab interno*, with the Nd:YAG laser) or externally (*ab externo*, with the holmium laser) to produce a direct opening into the anterior chamber through limbal tissue to achieve filtration. These laser procedures may be done using a probe (contact) or a contact lens (non-contact).

Indications

Laser sclerotomy may be considered for previously operated eyes, in which minimal or no conjunctival dissection is desired. However, for eyes without prior surgery, standard trabeculectomy is currently favored. The Nd:YAG for the *ab interno* approach and THC:YAG (holmium) for the *ab externo* approach have the most available clinical data. The holmium *ab externo* sclerotomy is generally more suitable for creating blebs in eyes with heavy conjunctival scarring that may severely limit the location of a repeat trabeculectomy, yet allow the passage of a laser probe. The Nd:YAG *ab interno* sclerotomy requires no conjunctival dissection, but because an instrument is passed across the anterior chamber, eyes should be aphakic or pseudophakic to avoid the risk of lens trauma.

Technique

Preparation

Depending on patient cooperation, the eye is anesthetized with subconjunctival, peribulbar, or retrobulbar anesthesia. A lid speculum is placed.

Ab externo technique: THC:YAG (Holmium)

Laser energy is delivered through a fiberoptic probe via a subconjunctival approach. The laser is set at a repetition rate of 5 pulses per second with an energy of 80–120 mJ per pulse. The eye is rotated inferiorly. A sclerotomy site is chosen either in the area with least conjunctival scarring or adjacent to a prior iridectomy. A 1–2 mm conjunctival incision is made about 8–10 mm away from the intended sclerotomy site and 6 mm from the limbus using Vannas scissors. The underlying Tenon's capsule is also incised until bare sclera is reached. The probe is then inserted under the Tenon's capsule and carefully advanced toward the limbus. It is manipulated into position at the limbus as anterior as possible without folding the conjunctiva under the probe. The aiming beam exits 90 degrees from the tip of the probe. With the probe tip held tangential to the limbus, the probe is rotated so that the aiming beam is as parallel as possible to the iris (Figure 12.7).

The conjunctiva over the probe tip is irrigated with balanced salt solution while the laser is fired. The surgeon is able to recognize sclerotomy patency by three signs: 1) small bubbles may appear in the anterior chamber; 2) the sound

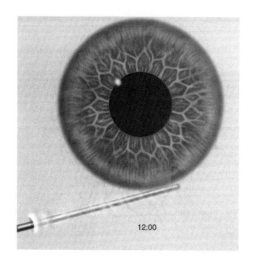

12:00

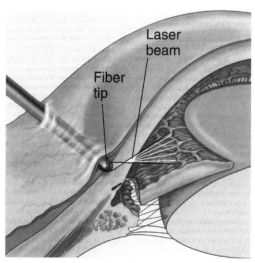

Fiber tip

Laser beam

Figure 12.7 Ab externo sclerotomy. The laser probe is advanced subconjunctivally and held tangential to the limbus (Above). The laser energy exits 90 degrees from the tip of the probe in a direction parallel to the iris, entering the anterior chamber. *Reproduced with permission from: Leen MM, Terebuh AK, Spaeth GL. Full thickness filtration surgery: incisional and laser techniques. In: Lindquist TD, Lindstrom RL (eds). Ophthalmic Surgery. Chicago: Mosby-Year Book Medical Publishers, 5th edn, 1996; Section III-H-14.*

of the laser ticking will change from a dull to a sharp noise; and 3) a bleb will form upon removal of the probe. The laser probe is then withdrawn and the conjunctival wound is closed with a running 8-0 vicryl suture. 5-fluorouracil can be injected subconjunctivally in an adjacent quadrant.

Ab interno technique: Nd:YAG

Laser energy is delivered through a fiberoptic probe via a transcameral approach. The laser is set at an energy of 200 mJ (10 W × 0.2 seconds).

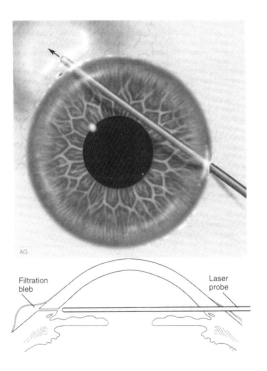

Figure 12.8 Ab interno sclerotomy. The laser probe is advanced through a corneal paracentesis and across the anterior chamber (Above). The laser energy exits along the long axis of the probe until the subconjunctival space is entered (Below). *Reproduced with permission from: Leen MM, Terebuh AK, Spaeth GL. Full thickness filtration surgery: incisional and laser techniques. In: Lindquist TD, Lindstrom RL (eds). Ophthalmic Surgery. Chicago: Mosby-Year Book Medical Publishers, 5th edn, 1996;Section III-H-17.*

Balanced salt solution or viscoelastic is injected subconjunctivally using a 30 gauge needle to elevate conjunctiva adjacent to the proposed sclerotomy site. A sharp steel blade or diamond knife is used to create a peripheral corneal paracentesis, about 1.5 mm in length, 90–180 degrees away from the proposed sclerotomy site. Viscoelastic is injected intracamerally through the paracentesis site. A vitrectomy instrument without infusion is used to create a peripheral iridectomy. The laser probe is introduced through the paracentesis and is passed across the anterior chamber until the tip is in contact with the sclera in the region of Schwalbe's line. A gonioscopy lens can be used to aid in visualization but is rarely needed.

The laser energy exits from the tip parallel to the long axis of the probe. Between 3 and 5 pulses are required to achieve filtration. The laser probe is advanced until the probe tip is visualized in the subconjunctival space (Figure 12.8). Penetration through full-thickness sclera is evident when an adjacent bleb enlarges. The probe is withdrawn. Additional balanced salt solution or viscoelastic is injected into the anterior chamber to verify the patency of the sclerostomy and further elevate the bleb. 5-fluorouracil (50 mg/ml, 5 mg) can be injected subconjunctivally in an adjacent quadrant.

197

Complications

Iris incarceration is the most frequent complication of ab externo laser filtration procedures, especially in phakic eyes and in those with narrow angles. The risk of this complication can be reduced by doing the sclerotomy over a prior peripheral iridectomy or by creating a peripheral iridectomy at the time of the sclerotomy. Postoperative iris prolapse can often be managed by massage over the sclerostomy site with a Zeiss gonioprism. Alternatively, a peripheral laser iridoplasty or laser iridotomy can be done. Other complications include hyphema, localized corneal edema, conjunctival burn or conjunctival buttonhole.

Laser sclerotomy procedures are also associated with those complications found in other full-thickness procedures. These include hypotony, shallow anterior chamber, choroidal effusion, choroidal hemorrhage, and cataract formation. Because minimal conjunctival manipulation helps to preserve episcleral tissue and increase the resistance to aqueous outflow, the occurrence of a shallow or flat anterior chamber may not be as common as would be expected for a full-thickness procedure.

Prognosis

The success rate of the holmium laser *ab externo* sclerostomy in 54–73% at 12 months, 36–52% at 2 years, and 36% at 4 years. A success rate for YAG laser *ab interno* sclerotomy of 60% at 2 years has been reported. These success figures primarily include eyes at high risk of filtration failure that also received adjunctive 5-fluorouracil. The role of laser sclerotomy in glaucoma filtration surgery as a primary or secondary procedure remains to be determined.

Suggested reading

Azuara-Blanco A, Dua HS. Malignant glaucoma after diode laser cyclophotocoagulation. *Am J Ophthalmol* 1999;**127**:467–9.

Dickens CJ, Nguyen N, Mora JS et al. Long-term results of noncontact transscleral neodymium:YAG cyclophotocoagulation. *Ophthalmology* 1995;**102**:1777–81.

Friedman DS, Katz LJ, Augsburger JJ, Leen M. Holmium laser sclerostomy in glaucomatous eyes with prior surgery: 24-month results. *Ophthalm Surg Lasers* 1998;**29**:17–22.

Glaucoma Laser Trial Research Group. The glaucoma laser trial (GLT) and glaucoma laser trial follow-up study: 7. results. *Am J Ophthalmol* 1995;**120**:718–31.

Iwach AG, Hoskins HD, Drake MV, Dickens CJ. Subconjunctival THC:YAG ('holmium') laser thermal sclerostomy. A one-year report. *Ophthalmology* 1993;**100**:356–65.

Kosoko O, Gaasterland DE, Pollack IP, Enger CL. Long-term outcome of initial ciliary ablation with contact diode laser transscleral cyclophotocoagulation for severe glaucoma. The Diode Laser Ciliary Ablation Study Group. *Ophthalmology* 1996;**103**:1294–302.

Meyer-Schwickerath G. Erfahrungen mit der lichtkoagulation der netzhaut und der iris. *Doc Ophthalmol* 1956;**10**:91–131.

Saunders DC. Acute angle closure glaucoma and Nd:YAG laser iridotomy. *Br J Ophthalmol* 1990;**74**:523–5.

Shields MB, Shields SE. Noncontact transscleral Nd:YAG cyclophotocoagulation: a long-term follow-up of 500 patients. *Trans Am Ophthalmol Soc* 1994;**92**:271–83.

Shingleton BJ, Richter CU, Belcher CD et al. Long-term efficacy of argon laser trabeculoplasty. *Ophthalmology* 1987;**94**:1513–8.

Spaeth GL, Baez KA. Argon laser trabeculoplasty controls one third of progressive, uncontrolled, open angle glaucoma for 5 years. *Arch Ophthalmol* 1992;**110**:491–4.

Tomey KF, Traverso CE, Shammas IV. Neodymium:YAG laser iridotomy in the treatment and prevention of angle closure glaucoma: a review of 373 eyes. *Arch Ophthalmol* 1987:**105**:476–81.

Wess HS, Shingleton BJ, Goode SM et al. Argon laser gonioplasty in the treatment of angle closure glaucoma. *Am J Ophthalmol* 1992;**114**:14–8.

Wilson RP, Javitt JC. Ab interno laser sclerostomy in aphakic patients with glaucoma and chronic inflammation. *Am J Ophthalmol* 1990;**110**:178–84.

13. GLAUCOMA SURGICAL PROCEDURES

Augusto Azuara-Blanco, Richard P Wilson, and Vital P Costa

Guarded filtration surgery or trabeculectomy

Trabeculectomy, or guarded filtration surgery, is the surgical procedure most commonly used to control intraocular pressure (IOP) in glaucomatous patients. Filtration surgery lowers the IOP by creating a fistula between the anterior chamber and the subconjunctival space. This leads to the accumulation of fluid below the conjunctiva, creating a filtering bleb (Figure 13.1).

Anesthesia

Retrobulbar, peribulbar or sub-Tenon's anesthesia is used in most cases. Topical anesthesia with a small subconjunctival injection of local anesthetic is becoming more popular. General anesthesia is usually reserved for children or non-cooperative patients.

Choosing the surgical site

Most authors prefer to do the first surgery at 12 o'clock as the filtration bleb is more likely to be covered by the superior eye-lid. This location would allow, if needed, two subsequent filtration surgeries in the superior conjunctiva (i.e. supero-nasal and supero-temporal). Inferior bleb positions are not recom-

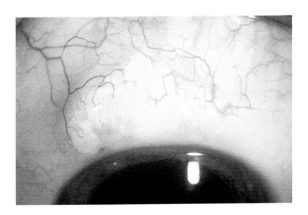

Figure 13.1
Appearance of a functioning filtering bleb.

mended, as the risk for the development of late endophthalmitis is markedly increased.

Fixation suture

A superior rectus traction suture (4-0 or 5-0 black silk on a tapered needle) rotates the globe inferiorly to bring the superior bulbar conjunctiva into view. Alternatively, a corneal traction suture in the quadrant of the planned surgery (7-0 or 8-0 black silk or nylon, or 6-0 or 7-0 Vicryl on a spatulated needle) can be used. The needle is passed through clear, midstromal cornea about 2 mm from the limbus for about 3–4 mm.

Conjunctival flap

A limbus- or fornix-based conjunctival flap is made with Wescott scissors and a non-toothed utility forceps. A fornix-based flap may be easier in cases with pre-existing perilimbal scarring and for combined cataract-filtration procedures.

When forming limbal-based flaps, the conjunctival incision is placed 8–10 mm posterior to the limbus (Figure 13.2). Once the conjunctiva is incised, the Tenon's capsule is grasped, raised, and cut with Wescott scissors. The conjunctival and Tenon's wound should be lengthened to about 10–14 mm cord length, with the Tenon's incision longer than the conjunctival incision because of the relative elasticity of the conjunctiva. During anterior dissection, the surgeon should grasp the Tenon's tissue rather than the conjunctiva to avoid an inadvertent buttonhole. The dissection is carried forward until the insertion of the Tenon's is reached, to clearly expose the corneoscleral limbus (Figure 13.2). In cases with extensive scarring from prior surgery, elevation of tissues with an injection of saline before dissection of the conjunctiva is useful to show scarring and to determine a favorable site for surgery.

When making fornix-based flaps, the conjunctiva and Tenon's are disinserted with a blade or Wescott scissors. An oblique relaxing incision at one or both corners can improve scleral exposure, especially if the conjunctiva is very thin. A 2 clock hour limbal peritomy (5–6 mm) is sufficient. Blunt dissection is carried out posteriorly using a blunt-tipped Wescott scissors, avoiding the superior rectus muscle.

The theoretical advantages of the fornix-based conjunctival flap may include improved exposure and access, reduced risk of conjunctival buttonhole formation, and the formation of a more posterior bleb. However, with a fornix-based flap there is an increased risk of conjunctival wound leak in the early postoperative period especially if antifibrosis agents are applied.

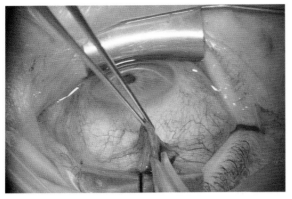

(A)

Figure 13.2
Trabeculectomy.
Surgical technique. A
limbal-based
conjunctival incision
is placed 8–10 mm
posterior to the
limbus (A) and
extended with
Wescott scissors (B).
The conjunctival
dissection is carried
forward to expose
the corneoscleral
limbus (C).

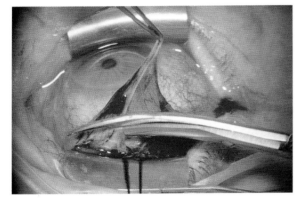

(B)

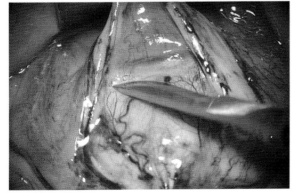

(C)

Scleral flap

The scleral flap should completely cover the sclerostomy to provide resistance to the aqueous outflow. The fluid will seep around the scleral flap into the subconjunctival space. Differences in the shape (rectangular, square, triangular, semicircular), or size of the scleral flap have little effect on surgical outcome. The determinants of outflow are the amount of overlap of the scleral flap over the inner trabeculectomy block, the number and tightness of the sutures holding down the scleral flap and, to a lesser extent, the thickness of the scleral flap.

After outlining the site of the scleral flap with cautery, the globe is fixated with toothed forceps and a blade is used to incise and dissect the scleral flap (Figure 13.3). The flap thickness should be between one-quarter and two-thirds of the scleral thickness. It is important to dissect the flap anteriorly (at least 1 mm into clear cornea) to ensure that the fistula is created anterior to the scleral spur and ciliary body. In eyes with angle closure glaucoma, peripheral

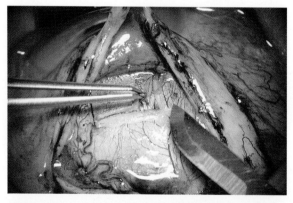

Figure 13.3
Trabeculectomy. Surgical technique. The scleral flap is outlined (A) and dissected into clear cornea (B).

(A)

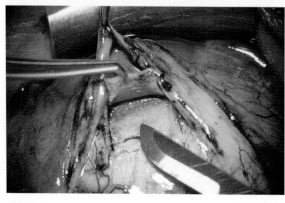

(B)

anterior synechiae, and/or small anterior segments, the flap dissection should be extended further anteriorly into the cornea.

Paracentesis track

A corneal paracentesis is made with a 27- or 30-gauge needle or a sharp-pointed blade before opening the globe. This is essential since it permits the surgeon to deepen and repressurize the anterior chamber during the procedure. The paracentesis is beveled to make the wound self-sealing, and aimed on entry into the inferior angle to reduce the chance of lens injury.

Internal block excision and peripheral iridectomy

A block of tissue at the corneoscleral junction is excised either with a super-sharp blade and Vannas scissors or with a punch (Figure 13.4). With the former technique, two radial incisions are made with a sharp blade starting in clear

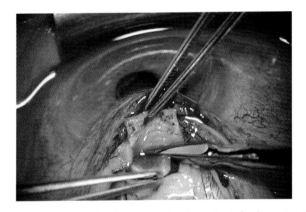

Figure 13.4
Trabeculectomy. Surgical technique. A block of tissue at the corneoscleral junction is excised with Vannas scissors.

cornea, at the most anterior point adjacent to the scleral flap, and extending posteriorly about 1–1.5 mm. The radial incisions are made about 2 mm apart. The blade or the Vannas scissors are used to connect the radial incisions, allowing the removal of a rectangular piece of tissue. Alternatively, the fistula can be created with a punch. An anterior corneal incision, parallel to the limbus, is made to enter into the anterior chamber, and a scleral punch is used to excise the limbal tissue. The fistula can be done close to one of the edges of the scleral flap to favor filtration in that direction.

A peripheral iridectomy is then done to prevent obstruction of the sclerectomy by the iris and to prevent postoperative pupillary block (Figure 13.5). The iris is grasped near its root with toothed forceps. The iris is retracted through the sclerostomy and a broad peripheral iridectomy is performed with Vannas or

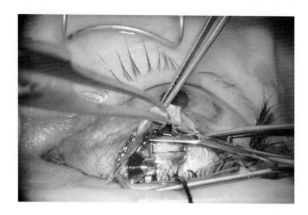

Figure 13.5
Trabeculectomy.
Surgical technique. A
peripheral
iridectomy is
performed with
Vannas scissors.

DeWecker scissors. The iridectomy should not extend too far posteriorly, to avoid iris root/ciliary body damage and bleeding.

Use of viscoelastic

In most cases, the use of viscoelastic is not necessary. A retentive viscoelastic may be advisable in eyes with high risk of aqueous misdirection or suprachoroidal hemorrhage (see below).

Closure of scleral flap

Releasable sutures

The scleral flap can be initially sutured with two interrupted 10-0 nylon sutures in rectangular flaps, and with an interrupted suture in triangular flaps (Figure 13.6). Slipknots are useful to adjust the tightness of the scleral flap and the rate of aqueous outflow. Additional sutures can be used to better control the outflow.

The surgeon can usually identify some 'key' sutures that appear to have more influence in restricting the aqueous outflow than others. These key sutures should be identified during surgery, when the anterior chamber is filled through the paracentesis and the flow around the scleral flap is observed. The key sutures should be identified in the patient's records so that the information is readily available postoperatively. Greater caution should be advised when releasing these 'key' sutures to increase the outflow.

Many surgeons prefer to reduce the risk of postoperative hypotony and anterior chamber shallowing by suturing the scleral flap to limit the flow of aqueous into the subconjunctival space to a barely visible ooze. Postoperatively, if the IOP is higher than desired, laser suture lysis can be used to lower the IOP in steps (Table 13.1). A tight suture closure may be more important in patients in whom the preoperative IOP is markedly raised, aphakic glaucomas, and

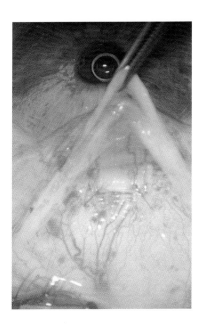

Figure 13.6 Trabeculectomy. Surgical technique. Two interrupted 10-0 nylon sutures have been used to secure the corners of the scleral flap.

patients at high risk of malignant glaucoma (i.e., chronic angle closure glaucoma), choroidal effusion and suprachoroidal hemorrhage (e.g. Sturge–Weber syndrome). In eyes with a postoperative subconjunctival hemorrhage, a krypton red or a diode laser should be used instead of an argon laser.

The use of releasable sutures allows the surgeon to close the scleral flap tightly, knowing that the flow can be increased postoperatively. Externalized releasable sutures are easily removed and do not require the use of laser equipment. They can be used in cases of inflamed or hemorrhagic conjunctiva or thickened Tenon's tissue (that would make suture lysis difficult).

Several surgeons have described different techniques. Among them are: Wilson (mattress-type suture with an externalized knot on the cornea), Shin (removable knot passed through the conjunctival bleb), Cohen and Osher (loop-

Table 13.1   Argon suture lysis

1. Argon laser parameters:
    spot size: 50–100 micron.
    exposure time: 0.02–0.1 sec (start with 0.05 sec).
    power: 500–800 mW (from 200 to 1000 mW).
2. Topical anesthesia (proparacaine 0.5%).
3. Contact lens (Hoskins, Ritch or other).
4. Focus the beam posterior to the conjunctiva.
5. If IOP still raised and bleb unchanged: gentle ocular massage or focal pressure.

knot suture externalized through the cornea), Hsu and Yarng (an externalized hemibow tie in the center of the filtering bleb), Maberley et al. (a two-arm 'U' suture that leaves no exposed suture end until one arm of the suture is removed), and Johnstone et al (releasable 'tamponade suture'). Releasable sutures are as effective as laser suture lysis. In theory, the disadvantages of releasable sutures include the need for additional intraoperative manipulation, possible postoperative discomfort from the externalized suture, corneal epithelial defects, and rarely, intraocular infection.

Intraoperative assessment of filtration

Using a 30-gauge cannula or needle, the anterior chamber can be reformed with balanced salt solution through the paracentesis track. Dry cellulose sponges are used to assess the adequacy of leakage around the scleral flap. The whole area is first dried and then the surgeon assesses the degree to which and rapidity with which the dry sponges become wet. This step is repeated, often many times, after adjusting the closure of the scleral flap. If flow seems excessive, or the anterior chamber shallows, the slipknots are tightened or additional sutures are placed. If aqueous does not flow through the flap, the surgeon may loosen the slipknots, replace tight sutures with looser ones or, alternatively, apply a cautery to the radial edges of the scleral flap, causing the wound to gape. The desired amount of flow is influenced by the diagnosis, severity of glaucomatous damage, preoperative IOP, and risk of hypotony-related complications.

Conjunctival closure

With limbus-based flaps, the Tenon's and conjunctiva layers can be closed separately with a double running suture using a 8-0 or 9-0 absorbable suture or,

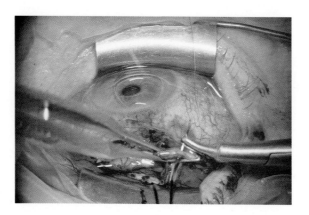

Figure 13.7
Trabeculectomy.
Surgical technique.
Closure of the
conjunctival incision.

alternatively, can be closed with a single layer using a 10-0 nylon running suture. A rounded-body needle is favored by many surgeons (Figure 13.7).

For conjunctival fornix-based flaps, some surgeons debride the peripheral corneal epithelium with a blade before suturing. Both conjunctival edges are positioned first making a tight conjunctiva/cornea apposition. Two 10-0 nylon sutures at the edges of the incision can be used to anchor the conjunctiva to the cornea, placing the sutures through midstromal peripheral cornea. Mattress sutures may be helpful, going through peripheral cornea, conjunctiva and returning through conjunctiva and cornea. When done, the relaxing incisions are also closed tightly (e.g. with running suture or in a purse string fashion) to ensure no unwanted leakage. After the wound is closed, a 30-gauge cannula is used to fill the anterior chamber with balanced salt solution through the paracentesis track to elevate the conjunctival bleb and to test for leaks.

Antibiotics and corticosteroids can be injected subconjunctivally into the inferior fornix. Alternatively, a collagen shield soaked in antibiotic-steroid solution can be used to cover the eye. Patching the eye depends on the patient's vision and the anesthesia used.

Prevention of filter failure

Topical steroids (e.g. prednisolone acetate 1%, 4–6 times daily) are routinely used postoperatively and tapered after 4–8 weeks. Antibiotics are required for 1–2 weeks after surgery. Postoperative cycloplegics (e.g. atropine 1% b.i.d or cyclopentolate 1% four times daily) may be used, especially in cases prone to shallow anterior chamber. If the anterior chamber is deep and there is no hypotony or inflammation, cycloplegics are not needed.

To further reduce postoperative subconjunctival fibrosis, especially in cases with a high risk of failure, adjunctive antifibrotic agents are used. Mitomycin-C and 5-fluorouracil (5-FU) inhibit fibroblast proliferation and subsequent scar tissue formation. Mitomycin C is 100 times more potent than intraoperative and postoperative 5-FU.

Because the use of antifibrotic agents is associated with higher success but also with higher complication rate, consideration of the risks and benefits should be made for each individual patient. One approach is to use mitomycin-C when one or more risk factors for failure concur, e.g. previous failed filtration procedure, aphakia/pseudophakia, previous conjunctival surgery, young patients, black race, uveitic glaucoma, and neovascular glaucoma. In primary filtration procedures without surgical risk factors, the use of antifibrotic agents depends on the surgeon's preference and characteristics of the patient (e.g. when a very low postoperative intraocular pressure is desired).

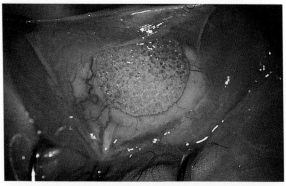

(A)

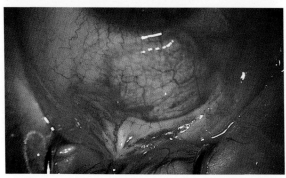

(B)

Figure 13.8
Trabeculectomy.
Surgical technique.
Intraoperative
application of
mitomycin-C with a
soaked filter paper
over the episclera
(A). The
conjunctival–Tenon's
layer is draped over
the sponge, avoiding
contact of the wound
edge with the
antifibrotic agent
(B).

Table 13.2 Subconjunctival injection of 5-fluorouracil (5-FU)
1. Confirm the absence of marked corneal epitheliopathy, bleb leak, and flat anterior chamber.
2. Topical anesthesia (e.g., proparacaine 0.5%); a cotton pledget can be soaked in anesthetic and applied to the area of injection. Topical antibiotic or povidone-iodine 5% solution.
3. A 30-G needle is attached to a 1 ml tuberculin syringe with the 5-FU.
4. Injection of 5 mg of 5-FU (0.1 ml, 50 mg/ml solution) subconjunctivally and 10 mm away from bleb.
5. Antibiotic ointment promptly applied after the injection.

Technique of intraoperative application of antimetabolites

Mitomycin-C (0.2–0.5 mg/ml solution) or 5-FU (25–50 mg/ml solution) can be applied for 1–5 minutes using a shaped, soaked cellulose sponge or filter paper over the episclera before dissecting the scleral flap (Figure 13.8). Some surgeons apply the antimetabolite under the scleral flap. The concentration and time of exposure vary according to the expected risk for fibrosis and the target IOP. The conjunctival–Tenon's layer is draped over the sponge, avoiding contact of the wound edge with the antifibrotic agent. After the application, the sponge is removed and the entire area is irrigated thoroughly with balanced salt solution (20–100 ml). The plastic devices that collect the liquid run-off are changed and disposed of according to toxic waste regulations.

In the postoperative period, subconjunctival 5-FU can be administered during the first postoperative days in 5 mg aliquots in cases prone to filtration failure (Table 13.2). The total number of injections is adjusted according to the function of the filtering bleb and the tolerance of the corneal epithelium. Complications associated with the use of postoperative 5-FU include corneal and conjunctival epithelial toxicity, corneal ulcers, conjunctival wound leaks, subconjunctival hemorrhage, or inadvertent intraocular spread of 5-FU. The frequency of complications is reduced with total dosages of 15–50 mg administered in 3–10 injections over the first 2–3 weeks.

Digital compression and focal compression

Digital ocular compression applied to the inferior sclera or cornea through the closed inferior eyelid, and focal compression with a moistened cotton-tip applicator at the edge of the scleral flap can be used to elevate the bleb and reduce the IOP in the early postoperative period, especially after laser suture lysis (Figure 13.9). This technique is not effective in cases of internal obstruction of the sclerostomy. When applying digital pressure, the patient is asked to look straight ahead while constant, moderate digital pressure is applied for 5–10 seconds over the cornea through the upper lid or over the inferior limbus through the lower lid. The bleb is then examined for changes in appearance (increased bleb height and area), and the IOP measured again. If there is complete occlusion of the trabeculectomy site, no reduction in IOP is seen and the bleb appears unchanged.

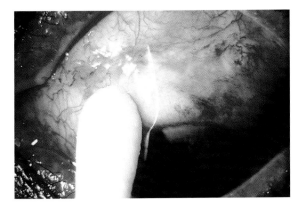

Figure 13.9 Focal compression with a moistened cotton tip applicator at the edge of the scleral flap (described by Carlo Traverso, MD) can increase outflow and reduce the IOP in the early postoperative period.

211

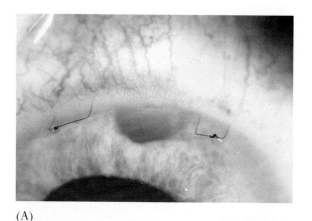

Figurea 13.10
Releasable suture
externalized through
the cornea,
described by one of
the authors, RPW
(A). Hoskins lens
and sutures treated
and cut with the
argon laser (B).

(A)

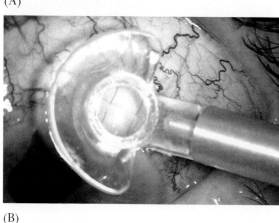

(B)

Timing of suture lysis or releasing sutures

This should be done when the function of the filtering bleb needs to be improved, ideally within the first 2 weeks after surgery when antimetabolites have not been used (Table 13.1); if done later, fibrosis of the scleral flap may halt any beneficial effect of this procedure (Figure 13.10). However, the window of opportunity is enlarged when antimetabolites have been used. Risk factors for hypotony should also be considered (see above). Before suture lysis, gonioscopy is done to confirm the presence of an open sclerostomy with no tissue or clot occluding its entrance.

Complications of filtration surgery

Tables 13.3–13.6 summarize the management of the most common complications of glaucoma filtration surgery.

212

Table 13.3 Prevention of intraoperative and postoperative complications of trabeculectomy

Complication	Prevention
1. Conjunctival buttonholes	Identify and avoid areas of scarring if possible; use non-toothed forceps and blunt dissection as much as possible.
2. Scleral flap disinsertion	Avoid thin scleral flaps.
3. Vitreous loss	Detect high-risk cases (high myopia, previous intraocular surgery, trauma, aphakia, subluxated lens). Consider pre-operative mannitol. In aphakic eyes, consider planned anterior vitrectomy. Create anterior fistula and avoid peripheral iridectomy in aphakes with no vitreous in the anterior chamber.
4. Hyphema	Create fistula anterior to the scleral spur; peripheral iridectomy must not include iris root and ciliary body.
5. Suprachoroidal hemorrhage	Detect high-risk cases (aphakia, glaucoma, vitrectomized, myopia, postoperative hypotony, arteriosclerosis, high blood pressure, bleeding disorders). Correct bleeding abnormalities; use mannitol; tighten scleral flap; use viscoelastic; counsel to avoid Valsalva maneuvers after surgery; treat hypotony.
6. Aqueous misdirection	Detect high-risk cases (angle closure glaucoma, small-hyperopic eyes). Minimize intraoperative shallowing of anterior chamber; use viscoelastic; large peripheral iridectomy; avoid overfiltration. Cautious suture lysis or cutting/pulling releasable sutures. Taper slowly cycloplegics.
7. Late bleb leak	Avoid the unnecessary use of antifibrotic agents.
8. Overfiltration	Avoid bleb and wound leaks; suture the scleral flap tightly; test filtration intraoperatively.
9. Flat anterior chamber	Avoid causes: overfiltration, choroidal effusion, suprachoroidal hemorrhage, aqueous misdirection, pupillary block. Anterior chamber maintainer suture in pseudophakic eyes.
10. Bleb encapsulation	Predisposing factors are male sex, glove powder, treatment with sympathomimetics, argon laser, or surgery.
11. Bleb failure	Intraoperatively: avoid tight scleral flap; consider antimetabolites; confirm the patency of the iridectomy. Postoperatively: early digital ocular massage or focal compression; suture lysis and cutting/pulling releasable sutures. Consider early 5-fluorouracil.

continued

213

Table 13.3 *continued*

Complication	Prevention
12. Corneal dellen	Related to abnormal tear film distribution with high bleb adjacent to cornea.
13. Hypotony maculopathy	Detect high risk cases: young and myopic patients. Cautious use of antimetabolites. Treat hypotony if visual acuity is reduced.
14. Cataract formation	Avoid intraoperative trauma. Treat flat anterior chamber and intense inflammation promptly. Avoid unnecessary steroids.
15. Blebitis, endophthalmitis	Patient education about early symptoms of infection. Prompt treatment of conjunctivitis/ blepharitis/red eye. Avoid soft contact lenses. Avoid inferior location for filtration procedures.

Table 13.4 Treatment of intraoperative and postoperative complications of trabeculectomy

Intraoperative complications	Treatment
1. Conjunctival buttonholes	Purse-string suture with 10-0 or 11-0 nylon on a tapered ('vascular') needle for central buttonholes. If the hole or tear occurs at the limbus or near the incision it can be sutured directly to the cornea or to the incision, respectively. A large bandage lens may be adequate to seal holes discovered in the postoperative period.
2. Scleral flap disinsertion	If sclerostomy has not been done, dissect a new scleral flap. If sclerostomy has been done, try to suture the flap into the limbal cornea with two horizontal mattress sutures. If not possible, use an autologous piece of Tenon's capsule or partial thickness sclera, or donor tissue (sclera, pericardium, fascia).
3. Vitreous loss	Automated anterior vitrectomy. Consider another trabeculectomy site.
4. Persistent bleeding	Cauterize source of hemorrhage.
5. Suprachoroidal hemorrhage	Prompt closure of eye, and gentle reposition of prolapsed uvea. Intravenous mannitol and acetazolamide (see also postoperative complications).

continued

214

Table 13.4 *continued*

Postoperative complications	Treatment
1. Hyphema	Initial observation and restriction of activity. Indication for surgical evacuation depends on IOP, size of hyphema, severity of optic nerve damage, likelihood of corneal staining, and presence of sickle-cell trait or anemia.
2. Suprachoroidal hemorrhage	Observation; control of IOP and pain. Drain 1 week after filtration surgery if the bleb or anterior chamber is flat or there is intolerable pain.
3. Aqueous misdirection	Initial medical treatment: intensive topical cycloplegic-mydriatic regimen, topical and oral aqueous suppressants, and osmotics. If possible, Nd:YAG laser hyaloidotomy (especially helpful in pseudophakic cases). Pars plana vitrectomy when previous therapies fail. In phakic eyes consider phacoemulsification, posterior capsulotomy and anterior vitrectomy.
4. Overfiltration	If anterior chamber is formed: cycloplegics, steroids, restriction in activity and avoidance of Valsalva maneuvers. If persists or if there is flat anterior chamber or visual loss, multiple options can be tried: large bandage contact lens, Simmon's shell, resuture scleral flap, cryotherapy, chemical irritants, argon laser, Nd:YAG thermal laser, autologous blood, surgical revision.
5. Choroidal effusions	Observation: cycloplegics, steroids. Drainage considered if no filtration by fourth postoperative day (bleb flat) or cornea endangered (Figure 13.11 and 13.12).
6. Flat anterior chamber	Treat cause (see Table 13.1). If there is lens–corneal touch, urgent reformation of the anterior chamber is necessary. If there are associated large choroidal effusions and a flat bleb, drainage of the fluid is advocated.
7. Bleb encapsulation	Initial observation. Aqueous suppressants if IOP is raised. Consider needling with 5-fluorouracil (Figure 13.13).
8. Bleb failure	*Early failure:* Identify mechanism. Clot in the internal ostium may need injection of tissue plasminogen activator (t-PA, 5 μg in 0.1 ml). External obstruction: digital ocular massage or focal compression; suture lysis and cutting/pulling releasable sutures; consider 5-fluorouracil. *Late failure:* In cases of episcleral fibrosis, external surgical revision or needling with 5-fluorouracil. In cases of internal obstruction of sclerostomy, Nd:YAG internal revision (Figure 13.14).

continued

Table 13.4 *continued*

Postoperative complications	Treatment
9. Corneal dellen	Artificial tears and ocular lubricants. Consider thermal Nd:YAG remodeling of limbal bleb (3 to 4 Joules with offset of 4 with Lasag, i.e. 1 to 1.3 mm below surface, with a desired end point of a white spot on the inner surface of the bleb, Figure 13.15).
10. Hypotony maculopathy	Treat cause (see above options to treat overfiltration/bleb leaks, Figures 13.16–13.19).
11. Late bleb leak	Several options: bandage contact lens, Simmon's shell, autologous blood, cryotherapy, thermal Nd:YAG laser, cyanoacrylate glue, fibrin tissue glue, surgical revision (Figures 13.20 and 13.21).
12. Cataract formation	Cataract extraction.
13. Blebitis, endophthalmitis	Stain and culture of samples (Figures 13.22 and 13.23).
	Bleb infection without intraocular involvement: intensive topical treatment with wide spectrum antibiotics.
	Bleb infection with anterior segment activity: intensive topical treatment with fortified antibiotics (e.g. cefazoline 50 mg/ml, and tobramycin 14 mg/ml).
	Bleb infection with vitreous involved: vitreous sample and intravitreal antibiotics are needed + topical fortified antibiotics. Consider PPV when visual acuity is severely reduced.

Table 13.5 Reformation of flat anterior chamber with viscoelastic

1. At the slit lamp or in the operating room. Topical anesthesia (e.g. tetracaine 0.5% or proparacaine 0.5%).
2. Topical antibiotic or povidone-iodine 5% solution.
3. Lid speculum (optional).
4. A 30-gauge needle (keeping air in the needle) is advanced through a corneal beveled tract starting near the limbus, and a small bubble of air followed by viscoelastic is injected into the anterior chamber.
5. End point: moderate deepening of the anterior chamber with IOP in 20s or low 30s.
6. Tonometry.
7. Topical antibiotics, cycloplegics and steroids.

Table 13.6   Needling of failing blebs

1. At the slit lamp or in the operating room.
2. Topical anesthesia (e.g. tetracaine 0.5% or proparacaine 0.5%); a cotton pledget can be soaked in anesthetic and applied to the area of injection. Topical antibiotic or povidone-iodine 5% solution.
3. Topical phenylephrine 2.5% to vasoconstrict the conjunctival vessels (optional).
4. A small volume of 2% lidocaine with epinephrine is injected around the bleb after landmarks are identified.
5. Lid speculum.
6. A 27-gauge needle or a MVR blade penetrates the conjunctiva as far as practical from the filtration site.
7. Needle (or blade) is advanced into the bleb cavity multiple times or the near and far wall of the scarred bleb is incised.
8. If required to raise a bleb, the needle or blade can be used to pierce through the thin scleral flap into the anterior chamber creating a small full-thickness filter (extreme caution in phakic eyes).
9. End point: elevation of the bleb + IOP reduction.
10. 10-0 nylon to close conjunctival entry wound if any leakage.
11. Topical antibiotics, cycloplegics and steroids.
12. Injection of 5-FU at the time of needling, and repeated 5-FU injections during the first 2 weeks after the procedure, increase the success rate dramatically.

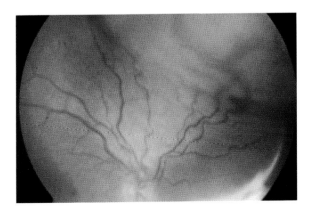

Figure 13.11
Choroidal effusion after filtration surgery. The IOP was 04 mmHg.

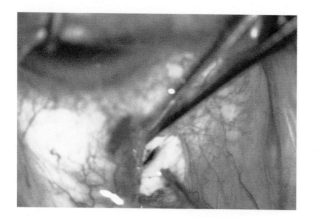

Figure 13.12
Drainage of
choroidal effusions.
A full-thickness
scleral incision is
made at least 4 mm
from the limbus.
Drainage of
choroidal effusions
should be combined
with infusion of
balanced salt solution
into anterior
chamber.

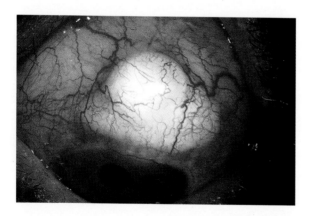

Figure 13.13
Encapsulated bleb,
highly vascularized,
elevated and with a
thick fibrotic bleb
wall.

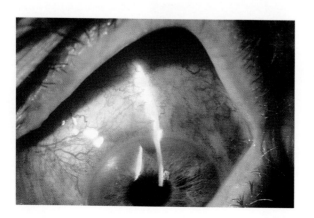

Figure 13.14 Flat,
failed filtering bleb.

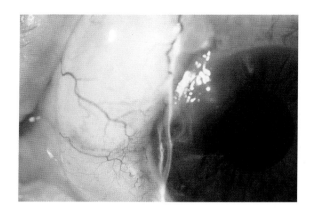

Figure 13.15
Corneal dellen caused by the elevated filtering bleb close to the cornea.

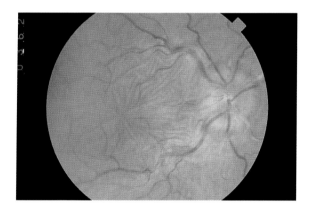

Figure 13.16
Hypotony maculopathy. Chorioretinal folds, tortuous vessels and edema of the peripapillary choroids are seen. The IOP was 05 mmHg.

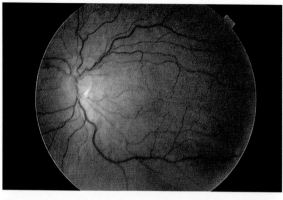

(A)

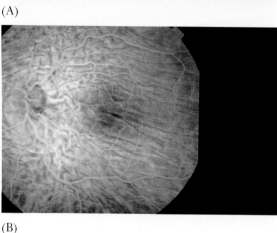

(B)

Figure 13.17
Hypotony maculopathy. This myopic patient underwent trabeculectomy without antifibrotic agents. Visual acuity before surgery was 20/20. After surgery, the IOP was 05–07 mmHg, and visual acuity was 20/200–20/400. On fundus examination, no clear abnormalities were seen (A). On fluorescein angiography, chorioretinal folds were detected (B).

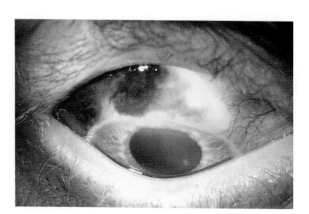

Figure 13.18
Autologous blood injection into the filtering bleb. This treatment can be used in patients with chronic hypotony related to overfiltration or late bleb leaks.

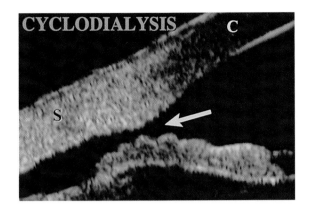

Figure 13.19
Ultrasound biomicroscopy of a patient with a cyclodialysis cleft after filtration surgery. The ciliary muscle is detached, and the aqueous humor flows directly to the suprachoroidal space.

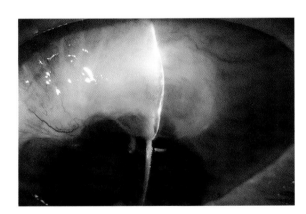

Figure 13.20
Thin, avascular, localized filtering bleb. This type of filtering bleb is likely to develop bleb leaks and blebitis.

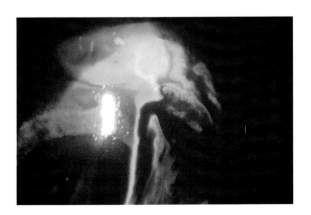

Figure 13.21
Seidel test (+) due to a late bleb leak.

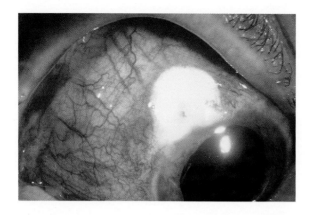

Figure 13.22 and 13.23 Bleb-related infection, 'blebitis'. There is an intense redness and loss of clarity of the filtering bleb. This severe complication can have devastating effects if the infection extends into the eye.

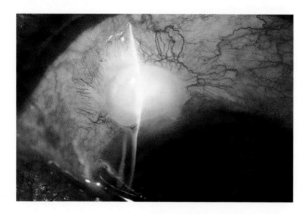

Aqueous misdirection (malignant glaucoma)

Aqueous misdirection (malignant glaucoma, ciliary block glaucoma) is characterized by shallowing of the anterior chamber without pupillary block or a suprachoroidal hemorrhage (Figure 13.24). Usually there is an accompanying rise in IOP. It occurs in 2–4% of patients operated on for angle closure glaucoma, but can occur after any type of incisional surgery. The chance of developing malignant glaucoma is greatest in phakic, hyperopic (small) eyes with angle closure glaucoma.

In this disorder, aqueous is diverted posteriorly into the vitreous cavity, increasing the vitreous volume and shallowing the anterior chamber. Decompression, shallowing of the anterior chamber, and the presence of a supra-

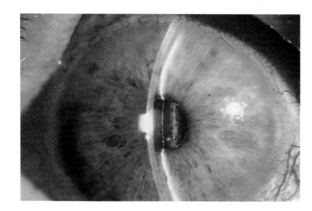

Figure 13.24:
Aqueous
misdirection
(malignant
glaucoma). A very
shallow anterior
chamber is seen. The
IOP was 49 mmHg.

ciliary effusion may precipitate ciliary block in predisposed eyes by inducing forward movement of the peripheral anterior hyaloid.

Aqueous misdirection usually occurs in the early postoperative period and is characterized by a shallow anterior chamber and high IOPs in the presence of a patent iridectomy. Indirect ophthalmoscopy and B-scan ultrasound confirm the absence of choroidal hemorrhage. If the adequacy of the surgical iridectomy is in doubt and pupillary block is possible, a laser iridotomy should be done.

Medical therapy, laser and vitreous surgery have been useful options in the treatment of aqueous misdirection. Medical treatment relieves about 50% of cases of aqueous misdirection. This condition is initially managed with mydriatic-cycloplegic drops, aqueous suppressants and hyperosmotics. Topical 1% atropine four times daily and 2.5% phenylephrine four times daily are used. These agents result in a posterior movement of the lens–iris diaphragm, allowing easier access of aqueous into the anterior chamber. Systemic carbonic anhydrase inhibitors and topical beta-adrenergic blocking agents at full dosage are important. Osmotics (isosorbide, glycerin, or intravenous mannitol) can also be very helpful in decreasing the fluid content of the vitreous cavity, and can be given every 8–12 hours. If medical treatment is well-tolerated and there are no contraindications, it can be maintained for 2–3 days. If the condition is relieved (i.e. the anterior chamber has deepened), hyperosmostic agents are discontinued first, and aqueous suppressants are reduced or even stopped over several days. Phenylephrine drops can be stopped, but the cycloplegic drops should be continued for months, or in some cases for years to prevent recurrence.

If medical therapy is unsuccessful and the ocular media are clear, a Nd:YAG laser capsulotomy and hyaloidotomy is used to disrupt the anterior vitreous face in pseudophakic and aphakic cases. The initial laser energy is between 2 and 4 millijoules, and the focus is placed posterior to the anterior hyaloid. After a successful Nd:YAG hyaloidotomy, a gradual deepening of the anterior chamber is usually seen. In pseudophakic eyes, a peripheral hyaloidotomy through the iridectomy is more efficient than a central hyaloidotomy because the lens capsule and intraocular lens can prevent communication between the vitreous cavity and the anterior chamber. In phakic eyes, phacoemulsification of the lens, rupture of posterior capsule and anterior vitrectomy can be considered. Pars plana vitrectomy should be considered when other therapies fail. A standard three-port pars plana vitrectomy, removing the anterior vitreous and part of the anterior hyaloid, is done. With the advent of pars plana vitrectomy, removal of a clear lens is rarely considered. Pars plana tube-shunt insertion with vitrectomy has been recommended for treatment of patients with aqueous misdirection, especially in cases with angle closure glaucoma. The implantation of the tube shunt through pars plana can help prevent recurrence of this disorder and can provide long-term control of IOP. In pseudophakic eyes, zonulo-hyaloido-vitrectomy via the anterior chamber can be performed.

Prevention: In high-risk eyes undergoing cataract or filtration surgery, hypotony and shallowing of the anterior chamber should be minimized. In filtration procedures, the use of intracameral viscoelastic and a large peripheral iridectomy can be helpful. Postoperative overfiltration should be avoided with a thick scleral flap sutured tighter and with more sutures than usual. A postoperative shallow anterior chamber due to overfiltration should be vigorously treated. Postoperatively, judicious suture lysis or cutting/pulling releasable sutures and slow tapering of cycloplegics are recommended.

Management of coexisting cataract and glaucoma

Combined surgery is usually indicated for patients with glaucomatous damage and cataract, whose IOP is uncontrolled or marginally controlled on two or more ocular hypotensive agents and whose cataract is visually significant or is likely to become so as a result of the intraocular surgery. Combined surgery is now usually preferable to sequential glaucoma and cataract procedures. However, when the glaucomatous damage is mild and IOP is controlled using only one or two topical medications, phacoemulsification alone through a corneal incision is recommended. On the other hand, in patients with advanced glaucomatous damage who require only one medication to control IOP, combined cataract/glaucoma surgery is advisable to reduce the risk of a postoperative IOP spike.

When performing combined procedures, phacoemulsification offers several advantages over extracapsular extraction. It preserves more conjunctiva for future filtering procedures, reduces the risk of intraoperative suprachoroidal hemorrhage, and promotes earlier visual rehabilitation.

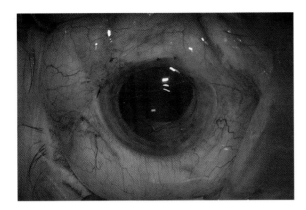

Figure 13.25
Combined
phacoemulsification
and trabeculectomy.
An elevated filtering
bleb is seen after
watertight closure of
the fornix-based
conjunctival incision,
at the end of the
procedure.

Combined phacoemulsification and trabeculectomy

Some surgeons do phacoemulsification through a temporal corneal incision and do a separate filtration procedure superiorly. Other surgeons use the same incision for both purposes. In the latter option, the combined surgery can be undertaken using either a fornix- or a limbus-based conjunctival flap in the superior limbus. Mitomycin-C and 5-FU (applied before the scleral flap is dissected) may improve the success rate of filtration surgery when it is associated with cataract extraction, and are recommended.

Different shapes of scleral flap can be used. Some surgeons use a standard scleral tunnel incision and fashion the sides of the flap after the phacoemulsification of the lens is completed. After the partial-thickness scleral flap is done, a 3.0 keratome is advanced under the sclera and used to enter into the anterior chamber in a dimpling-down maneuver. This completes a triplanar incision, which provides wound stability. Phacoemulsification is then done, and a foldable intraocular lens is inserted. There is no evidence for the superiority of any type of posterior chamber intraocular lens in combined procedures, but it is thought that the smaller incisions used for foldable lenses produce less postoperative inflammation and astigmatism.

After the insertion of the intraocular lens, a block of corneal–trabecular tissue is removed with a scleral punch (see above). This is followed by aspiration of viscoelastic and a peripheral iridectomy. The scleral flap is then sutured with 10-0 nylon sutures to control the aqueous outflow, allowing a slow ooze of aqueous. The conjunctiva/Tenon wound is sutured watertight, and subconjunctival steroids and antibiotics are applied to the eye (Figure 13.25).

Combined extracapsular cataract extraction and trabeculectomy

This technique is used only in exceptional circumstances. A fornix-based conjunctival incision provides better and easier access to the surgical site.

225

Antifibrotic agents can be applied before the scleral flap for the filtration procedure is fashioned, usually at the center of the cataract incision. A partial-thickness limbo-scleral groove is then extended on either side of the scleral flap, and then the dissection is carried out about 1 mm anteriorly. A paracentesis is made, and the anterior chamber is also entered through the limbo-scleral groove. This latter incision is used to do a standard capsulotomy, hydrodissection and lens manipulation. Then, corneoscleral scissors or a sharp blade are used to extend the limbo-scleral incision across the preformed groove and the anterior part of the scleral flap to an adequate width. The lens nucleus and cortex are removed in the usual fashion, followed by implantation of an intraocular lens. The portion of the limbo-scleral wound outside the scleral flap is then closed with 10-0 nylon, and a block of corneal–trabecular tissue is removed from under the scleral flap. This is followed by aspiration of viscoelastic and a peripheral iridectomy. The scleral flap is then sutured with 10-0 nylon sutures to control the aqueous outflow, allowing a slow ooze of aqueous.

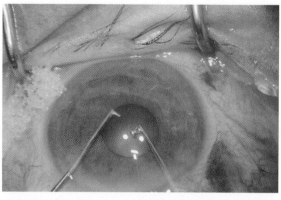

(A)

Figure 13.26
Combined phacoemulsification and trabeculectomy. Pupillary stretching with two collarbutton retractors. The retractors engage the iris sphincter (A) and stretch the pupil toward the anterior chamber angle in opposite directions (B).

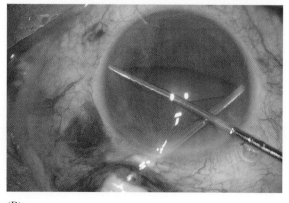

(B)

226

The peripheral corneal epithelium is debrided with a blade and the conjunctiva is sutured at the corners under tension, with some overlap of the conjunctiva onto the cornea. A continuous or central mattress 10-0 nylon suture is used to secure the conjunctival wound.

Management of the small pupil

A properly dilated pupil is important to avoid complications of cataract surgery. Patients who have used miotics may not have adequate pupil dilation, and there are several options to allow cataract surgery.

Pupillary stretching with two iris hooks or collarbutton retractors is easy and quick (Figure 13.26). The hooks or retractors engage the iris sphincter and stretch the pupil toward the anterior chamber angle in opposite directions. The maneuver is repeated in different meridians until the pupil reaches adequate size. Multiple sphincterotomies quickly enlarge the pupil but may increase postoperative inflammation (Figure 13.27). Stern-Gills, Vannas or other fine scissors are employed to make multiples cuts to the iris's sphincter of about 0.5 mm in length. Flexible iris hooks (Grieshaber hooks) are preferred by many surgeons but are expensive. From two inferior to four equally spaced hooks around the limbus are introduced through peripheral corneal paracentesis tracts in each quadrant. After they engage the pupil, each hook is retracted to the desired position and the silicone sleeve is displaced anteriorly against the cornea to retain the hooks in position. Lastly, the Grether pupil expander can be also used. This device is introduced into the eye with an inserter and includes three iris hooks that engage the iris sphincter, expanding it.

Glaucoma drainage devices

Glaucoma drainage devices (GDD), also called aqueous shunts or tube shunts, are an alternative surgical treatment in eyes with poor surgical prognosis for guarded filtration surgery. Modern aqueous shunting procedures were introduced in 1969 by Molteno, who used a posteriorly placed episcleral bleb-promoting implant (Figure 13.28) connected to a segment of silicone tubing, which was inserted into the anterior chamber (Figure 13.29). There are now several devices available, which differ in the presence or absence of a flow-limiting element and the design of the episcleral plate or plates.

Indications

The use of a GDD is indicated in patients with uncontrolled glaucoma in whom filtration surgery with antifibrotic agents has already failed or is unlikely to

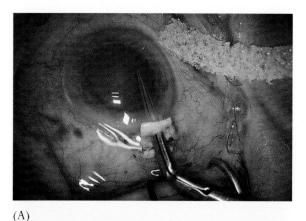

Figure 13.27
Combined
phacoemulsification
and trabeculectomy.
Multiple
sphincterotomies
about 0.5 mm long
allow enlargement of
the pupil (A and B).

(A)

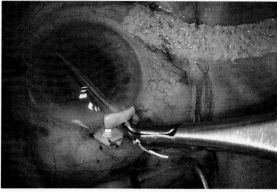

(B)

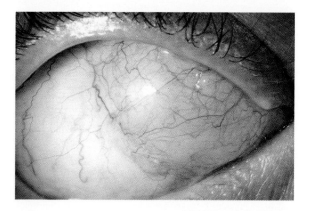

Figure 13.28
Glaucoma drainage
device. Posterior
encapsulation
surrounding the
explant.

succeed. There is now an increasing role for shunting procedures in the management of advanced congenital and juvenile glaucoma, traumatic glaucoma, aphakic and pseudophakic glaucoma, postkeratoplasty glaucoma and other secondary

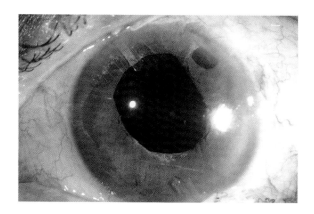

Figure 13.29
Glaucoma drainage
device. Silicone tube
in the anterior
chamber.

glaucomas. Primary implantation of a shunt device may be advised in eyes with neovascular glaucoma, extensive perilimbal scarring or anteriorly located synechiae.

In some cases, vitreoretinal surgery may be combined with tube shunt implantation through pars plana, especially in eyes with neovascular glaucoma and vitreous haemorrhage (associated with endolaser-photocoagulation) or in some aphakic or pseudophakic glaucomas, where vitreous may occlude the tube postoperatively.

Types of drainage devices

Implant designs fall into one of two categories based on the presence or absence of the element that limits aqueous flow through the anterior chamber tube.

Non-restrictive devices

These (e.g. Molteno, Schocket, Baerveldt) permit the free flow of fluid from the inner ostium of the tube in the anterior chamber to the episcleral explant.

Restrictive devices

These (e.g. Krupin, Joseph, White, Optimed, Ahmed) incorporate an element in the posterior part of the tube (i.e. valve, membrane, or resistant matrix), designed to limit fluid flow to prevent postoperative hypotony. In addition, the size, shape, and material used for the episcleral plate differ among the various implants (Table 13.7). The devices are made of materials to which fibroblasts cannot firmly adhere (polypropylene, polymethylmethacrylate, silicone).

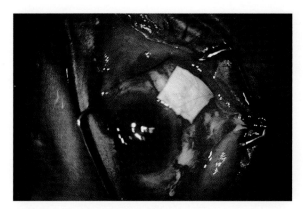

Figure 13.32 Glaucoma drainage device. Surgical technique. Donor sclera is used to cover the limbal portion of the tube. The patch graft is sutured in place using interrupted nylon sutures.

anterior chamber with smooth forceps. Proper positioning of the tube in the anterior chamber is essential, ensuring that it does not touch the iris, lens, or cornea. The last two steps should be repeated if the tube is not ideally placed into the anterior chamber, or if the length of the tube is not adequate. The tube is fixed to the sclera with sutures of 10-0 nylon or prolene. The anterior suture is wrapped tightly around the tube to prevent movement into or out of the anterior chamber. To avoid postoperative conjunctival erosion of the tube, donor sclera, fascia lata, dura mater or pericardium are used to cover the limbal portion of the tube (Figure 13.32). The patch graft is sutured in place using interrupted nylon sutures, with the knots rotated onto the episclera.

During the insertion of *non-restrictive devices*, an additional step is needed to prevent postoperative hypotony. This step should be made before suturing the plate to episclera. The tube can be occluded by placing a 4-0 or 5-0 nylon suture (Latina suture) into the tube from the reservoir side, with enough suture coming out of the tube to place its other end subconjunctivally in the inferior quadrant. The tube is then ligated with an absorbable 6-0 to 8-0 Vicryl suture depending upon the period of time desired until the tube becomes functional. If the pressure cannot be controlled with medication during the period before the ligature dissolves, a small cut in the inferior conjunctiva far away from the reservoirs allows the nylon suture to be pulled from the tube lumen, making the shunt functional. Another option is to ligate the tip of the tube with a 10- or 9-0 prolene suture that can be expanded by warming with the Argon laser (0.5 W, 0.5 sec.). Since the tube is completely ligated, several venting slits in the anterior extrascleral portion of the tube can be made with a sharp 15-degree blade or by passing the needle on the 6-0 Vicryl suture through the tube to allow some aqueous outflow in the early postoperative period. The amount of aqueous egress can be checked with a 27-gauge cannula on a syringe with saline inserted into the end of the tube.

When pars plana vitrectomy is associated with tube–shunt implantation, the shunt reservoir(s) is prepared and sutured to the episclera before vitrectomy. At the end of the vitrectomy, the tube is inserted through a 22-gauge needle track in pars plana. The appropriate position and length of the tube within the posterior segment should be confirmed in the operating room. The length of tube required is longer than expected, and the tip of the tube should be seen at the edge of the pupil without the aid of a gonioscope. A watertight conjunctival closure is essential and is accomplished in the same manner as a trabeculectomy or combined cataract–trabeculectomy.

Postoperative care

The postoperative regimen includes a topical antibiotic and cycloplegic for 2–4 weeks, and topical steroids for 2–3 months postoperatively. Antiglaucoma medication is added as required to achieve adequate IOP reduction.

In *non-restrictive devices*, the stent suture is removed 4–6 weeks after surgery, or sooner in the early postoperative period if the IOP is dangerously raised despite antiglaucoma medications. At the slit-lamp, under topical anesthesia, a 1–2 mm conjunctival incision is made above the suture end, which is then slowly pulled from the tube lumen. It is unnecessary to suture this wound.

Results

The highest success rates with GDD have been achieved in eyes with open- or closed-angle glaucoma, either phakic or aphakic/pseudophakic, and in eyes that previously failed filtration surgery. Success is usually lowest in eyes with neovascular glaucoma. After GDD, visual acuity is maintained within one line of preoperative acuity in most patients, although the visual outcome of patients with neovascular glaucoma is primarily determined by the underlying disease.

The Molteno implant is probably the most widely used device and has been in use for more than 20 years. Reports using either a single-plate or double-plate Molteno implant indicate a success rate of between 60% and 90% after at least 6 months' follow-up, and a lower success rate in cases with neovascular glaucoma (from 22% to 67%). The level of IOP may be directly related to the area of the episcleral plate and to the area of the bleb. Double-plate devices control IOP better than single-plate implants, probably due to the larger surface area. However, 350 mm^2 Baerveldt devices appear to have better outcome than 500 mm^2 Baerveldt explants.

Complications

Implantation of aqueous tube shunts is associated with a significant risk of postoperative complications. Early postoperative complications include hypotony, flat anterior chamber, choroidal effusions, suprachoroidal hemorrhage (Figure 13.33), aqueous misdirection, hyphema, and increased IOP. Hypotony, the most common complication, is usually due to excessive outflow of aqueous humor. It may result in a flat anterior chamber and choroidal detachment (Figure 13.34). Recurrent flat anterior chamber may require additional tube ligation. Restrictive or valved implants may be less commonly complicated with hypotony than non-restrictive devices.

High IOP can be related to occlusion of the tube by fibrin, a blood clot, iris or vitreous. Fibrin or blood may resolve spontaneously, however, an intracameral injection of tissue plasminogen activator helps to dissolve the clot within a few hours. When the iris tissue occludes the lumen of the tube, Nd:YAG laser iridotomy or argon laser iridoplasty may re-establish the patency of the tube. Vitreous incarceration can be treated successfully with Nd:YAG laser, but an

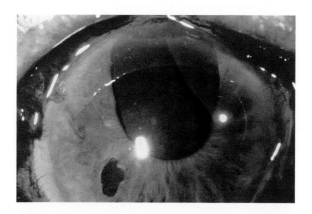

Figure 13.33
Glaucoma drainage device. Massive suprachoroidal hemorrhage in an aphakic patient after a Molteno implantation.

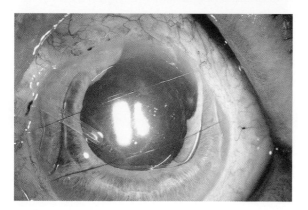

Figure 13.34
Glaucoma drainage device. To prevent flat anterior chamber, an anterior chamber maintainer suture (10-0 prolene) can be used in pseudophakic eyes, especially in eyes with high risk of complications.

234

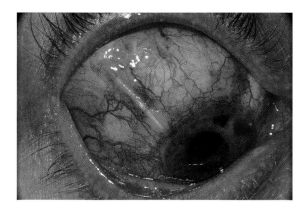

Figure 13.35
Glaucoma drainage
device. Melting of
pericardial patch
graft and
conjunctival erosion.

anterior vitrectomy may be necessary to prevent recurrence. The tube can also
retract from the anterior chamber. If the tube is too short (i.e. not seen in the
anterior chamber), the tube may be lengthened by splicing another piece of
tubing with the aid of a coupling segment of angiocath.

Late postoperative complications of aqueous shunting procedures include increased
IOP, hypotony, implant migration, conjunctival erosion (Figure 13.35), corneal edema
or decompensation, cataract, diplopia, and endophthalmitis. Late failure with
increased IOP can be caused by blockage of the anterior chamber tube opening (see
above) and, most commonly, by excessive fibrosis around the plate. Surgical bleb
revision (excision or needling of the fibrous wall) with antifibrosis agents can be
helpful. A failed procedure can also be managed by implantation of additional aqueous
shunts. Corneal decompensation may result from direct contact between the tube and
the cornea. When there is tube–cornea touch, repositioning of the tube should be
considered, especially in cases where there is the risk of endothelial failure (i.e. cases
with focal corneal edema, or after penetrating keratoplasty). Diplopia is caused by
mechanical restriction of the extraocular muscles. If diplopia is persistent and not
responsive to prisms, the shunt may need to be removed or relocated.

Cyclocryotherapy

Cyclocryotherapy lowers the IOP by destroying the epithelial and capillary
elements of the ciliary processes, resulting in decreased aqueous production.
Cyclocryotherapy was the cyclodestructive procedure of choice until the development of laser cyclophotocoagulation (see Chapter 12 on laser treatment).
Cyclocryotherapy is presently used where cyclophotocoagulation is not available,
or when the risk of sympathetic ophthalmia, which is seen rarely with cyclophotocoagulation but not cyclocryotherapy, is deemed unacceptable by the patient
or doctor. Cyclocryotherapy is reserved for patients with refractory glaucomas

and poor visual potential, and for pain reduction in eyes with absolute glaucoma.

In adult cooperative patients, the procedure is done under retrobulbar or peribulbar anesthesia. If the visual potential of the eyes treated is poor, a retrobulbar injection of absolute alcohol is used to anesthetize the eye for the first few postoperative months. After the retrobulbar local anesthetic is injected, the syringe is disengaged from the retrobulbar needle and the needle left in place until the block is effective. Then 0.5 cc of absolute alcohol is injected through the retrobulbar needle.

A nitrous oxide cryounit with a cryoprobe tip of 2.5–3.5 mm diameter is typically used. As the location of the ciliary body varies markedly between myopes and hyperopes, the location of the cryoprobe is directed by transillumination which reveals the dark band of the ciliary body. Typically, the anterior edge of the probe is placed 1–1.5 mm posterior from the limbus (Figure 13.36). The cryoprobe tip temperature should be –80°C, and each application should last 50 seconds for non-neovascular glaucomas and 60 seconds for neovascular

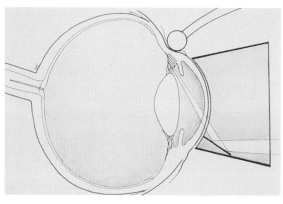

(A)

Figure 13.36
Cyclocryotherapy.
Surgical technique.
The anterior edge of
cryoprobe tip is
placed 1–1.5 mm
posterior from the
limbus (A and B).
Each application
should last 50–60
seconds.

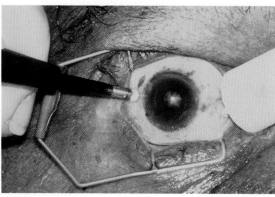

(B)

236

glaucomas. The ice ball may extend 1 to 2 mm into the peripheral cornea. One application is given at eight evenly distributed loci around the limbus or, alternatively, 180 confluent degrees of the ciliary body may be treated. If IOP increase is not severe and some functioning outflow is present, 3 or 4 clock hours can be treated. At the end of the operation, a subconjunctival injection of deposteroid is given, and atropine drops or ointment is instilled in the eye. All glaucoma medications except miotics and prostaglandins are continued, and frequent topical steroids and q.i.d. atropine are prescribed. If retrobulbar alcohol is used, oral tylenol is usually the only pain medication required.

If additional cryotherapy is needed, it should be done no sooner than 1 month after the initial procedure. If 360 degrees of treatment were originally administered, then eight loci over 360 degrees are again treated without shifting from the original treatment areas. If 180 degrees were treated, the second 180 degrees of treatment can be placed over one of the untreated quadrants and over one of the previously treated quadrants. The procedure can be repeated as needed.

Possible complications of cyclocryotherapy include severe pain, increase of IOP, hyphema (common in eyes with neovascular glaucoma), visual loss ('wiping out' fixation in patients with advanced optic nerve damage), choroidal detachment, retinal detachment, chronic hypotony, cystoid macular edema, anterior segment necrosis, vitreous hemorrhage, aqueous misdirection, cataract, lens subluxation, and phthisis bulbi. A major concern is the possibility of phthisis (about 8% at 1 year and 12% at 4 years), which is more common in patients with neovascular glaucoma.

Surgical procedures for congenital glaucoma

Goniotomy and trabeculotomy produce similar results. Goniotomy has the advantage of preserving the conjunctiva for possible future filtering surgeries, but cannot be done in cases with corneal clouding. In the latter cases, trabeculotomy is indicated.

Goniotomy

Goniotomy consists of an incision through the membrane holding the iris anteriorly, covering the trabecular meshwork. It is done under direct visualization with an operating microscope and a gonioscopy lens. The goniolens is placed on the nasal cornea, leaving about 2 mm of temporal cornea exposed for the knife entry. A paracentesis is made temporally beveling through the limbus well into clear cornea to prevent later anterior synechiae (Figure 13.37). Viscoelastics are then injected into the anterior chamber and a non-tapered goniotomy knife (or a 23-gauge needle) is then passed through the paracentesis and across the anterior chamber to the opposite angle. The blade is subsequently swept 120 to

237

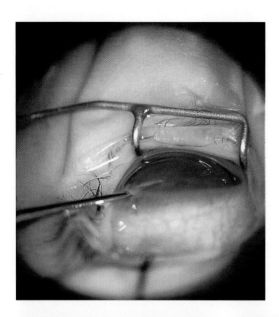

Figure 13.37
Goniotomy technique. The goniotomy knife is introduced into the anterior chamber. Fig. 13.37 Reproduced with permission from Traverso CE. Treatment of developmental glaucoma. In: Choplin NT, Lundy DC, eds. Atlas of Glaucoma. London; Martin Dunitz, 1998).

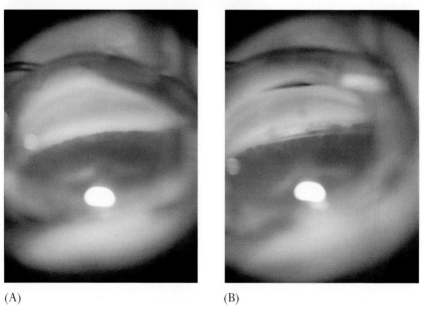

(A)   (B)

Figure 13.38 Goniotomy technique. Intraoperative gonioscopic view before (A) and immediately after goniotomy (B). Fig. Reproduced with permission from Traverso CE. Treatment of developmental glaucoma. In: Choplin NT, Lundy DC, eds. Atlas of Glaucoma. London; Martin Dunitz, 1998.

160 degrees just anterior to the iris insertion. The incision cuts only the abnormal tissue covering the trabecular meshwork. As the incision is made, the iris dramatically falls posterior, revealing a deep angle recess (Figure 13.38). An assistant rotates the eye clockwise and counterclockwise, with the eye stabilized by fixation sutures or locking forceps grasping the superior and inferior rectus muscles to extend the treated angle. The paracentesis track is then sutured and the viscoelastic is diluted or aspirated and replaced by balanced salt solution. Alternatively, attention can be turned to the nasal limbus and the procedure repeated on the other 180 degrees of angle.

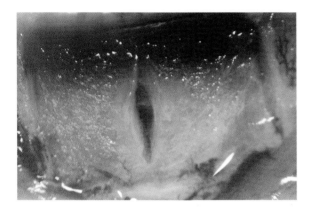

Figure 13.39 Trabeculotomy technique. Underneath the scleral flap, a radial incision is made until a change in the pattern of the connective fibers is seen, indicating the location of Schlemm's canal. Reproduced with permission from Traverso CE. Treatment of developmental glaucoma. In: Choplin NT, Lundy DC, eds. Atlas of Glaucoma. London; Martin Dunitz, 1998.

Trabeculotomy

Trabeculotomy begins with the dissection of a fornix- or limbal-based conjunctival flap and the creation of a partial thickness scleral flap hinged at the limbus.

A radial cut at the gray-white limbus transitional zone is then gradually deepened until the Schlemm's canal is identified (Figure 13.39). A trabeculotome is inserted fully into each end of Schlemm's canal and rotated into the anterior chamber, rupturing the trabecular meshwork (Figures 13.40 and 13.41). The parallel arm of the trabeculotomy serves as a guide. Alternatively, a 5-0 or 6-0 nylon or prolene suture can be threaded into Schlemm's canal for 360 degrees (Figure 13.42). Occasionally, Schlemm's canal cannot be identified and conversion to a filtering procedure is necessary.

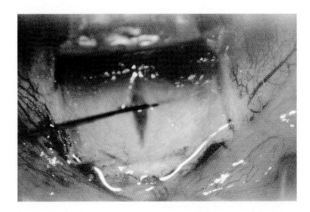

Figure 13.40 Trabeculotomy technique. The lower arm of a Harms' trabeculotome is introduced into Schlemm's canal. Reproduced with permission from Traverso CE. Treatment of developmental glaucoma. In: Choplin NT, Lundy DC, eds. Atlas of Glaucoma. London; Martin Dunitz, 1998.

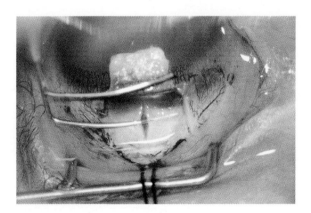

Figure 13.41 Trabeculotomy technique. The handle of the trabeculotome is rotated and the lower arm is pushed forward through the trabecular tissue into the anterior chamber. Reproduced with permission from Traverso CE. Treatment of developmental glaucoma. In: Choplin NT, Lundy DC, eds. Atlas of Glaucoma. London; Martin Dunitz, 1998.

Mild bleeding into the anterior chamber is usually noted. The scleral flap is then sutured into place, and the conjunctiva is closed in the same manner as for filtering procedures. Low-dose pilocarpine is used to keep the iris from adhering to the incised filtration angle.

240

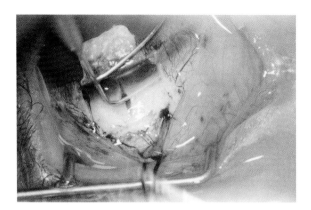

Figure 13.42 Trabeculotomy technique. Schlemm's canal is probed with a 6-0 nylon suture. Reproduced with permission from Traverso CE. Treatment of developmental glaucoma. In: Choplin NT, Lundy DC, eds. Atlas of Glaucoma. London; Martin Dunitz, 1998.

Severe complications with trabeculotomy and goniotomy are rare. Moderate bleeding into the anterior chamber is common. Blood clots usually resorb within a few days. Intraoperative complications during trabeculotomy are often related to the difficulty in identifying Schlemm's canal. This is more difficult in newborns and in eyes with anterior segment anomalies. The initial goal is to open the outer wall of Schlemm's canal without perforating the inner wall into the anterior chamber. If penetration into the anterior chamber occurs, the iris may prolapse. In that case, an iridectomy may be necessary. If the supraciliary space is wrongly probed, forward rotation into the anterior chamber is not possible unless considerable force is exerted, causing cyclodialysis and iridodialysis. If the tip of the trabeculotomy probe is held toward the cornea during rotation, a Descemet's membrane tear can occur. Usually these are small and rarely cause corneal edema.

Suggested reading

Addicks EM, Quigley HA, Green WR et al. Histologic characteristics of filtering blebs in glaucomatous eyes. *Arch Ophthalmol* 1983;**101**:795–8.

Azuara-Blanco A, Katz LJ, Gandham SB, Spaeth GL. Pars plana tube insertion of aqueous shunt with vitrectomy in malignant glaucoma. *Arch Ophthalmol* 1998;**116**:808–10.

Azuara-Blanco A, Katz LJ. Dysfunctional filtering blebs. *Surv Ophthalmol* 1998;**43**: 93–126.

Britt MT, LaBree LD, Lloyd MA et al. Randomized clinical trial of the 350-mm² versus the 500-mm² Baerveldt implant: longer term results: is bigger better?. *Ophthalmology* 1999;**106**:2312–8.

Chen C-W. Enhanced intraocular pressure controlling effectiveness of trabeculectomy by local application of MMC. *Trans Asia-Pacific Acad Ophthalmol* 1983;**9**:172.

Costa VP, Katz LJ, Spaeth GL et al. Primary trabeculectomy in young adults. *Ophthalmology* 1993;**100**:1071–6.

Costa VP, Moster MR, Wilson RP et al. Effects of topical mitomycin C on primary trabeculectomies and combined procedures. *Br J Ophthalmol* 1993;**77**:693–7.

Costa VP, Smith M, Spaeth GL et al. Loss of visual acuity after trabeculectomy. *Ophthalmology* 1993;**100**:599–612.

Costa VP, Spaeth GL, Eiferman RA et al. Wound healing modulation in glaucoma filtration surgery. *Ophthalmic Surg* 1993;**24**:152–70.

Costa VP, Wilson RP, Moster MR et al. Hypotony maculopathy following the use of topical mitomycin C in glaucoma filtration surgery. *Ophthalmic Surg* 1993;**24**:389–94.

Epstein DL, Steinert RF, Puliafito CA. Neodymium:YAG laser therapy to the anterior hyaloid in aphakic malignant (ciliovitreal block) glaucoma. *Am J Ophthalmol* 1984;**98**:137–43.

Gandham SB, Costa VP, Katz LJ et al. Aqueous tube-shunt implantation and pars plana vitrectomy in eyes with refractory glaucoma. *Am J Ophthalmol* 1993;**116**:189–95.

Gianoli F, Schnyder CC, Bovey E, Mermoud A. Combined surgery for cataract and glaucoma: phacoemulsification and deep sclerectomy compared with phacoemulsification and trabeculectomy. *J Cataract Refract Surg* 1999;**25**:340–6.

Heuer DK, Lloyd MA, Abrams DA et al. Which is better? One or two? A randomized clinical trial of single-plate versus double-plate Molteno implantation for glaucomas in aphakia and pseudophakia. *Ophthalmology* 1992;**99**:1512–9.

Jacobi PC, Dietlein TS, Krieglstein GK. Glaucoma triple procedure to treat pseudoexfoliation. *Arch Ophthalmol* 1999;**117**:1311–8.

Jay JL, Allan D. The benefit of early trabeculectomy versus conventional management in primary open-angle glaucoma relative to severity of disease. *Eye* 1989;**3**:528–35.

Johnson DH. Options in the management of malignant glaucoma. *Arch Ophthalmol* 1998;**116**:799–800.

Kim YY, Sexton RM, Shin DH et al. Outcomes of primary phakic trabeculectomies without versus with 0.5- to 1-minute versus 3- to 5-minute mitomycin C. *Am J Ophthalmol* 1998;**126**:755–62.

Kitazawa Y, Matsushita HS, Yamamoto T et al. Low-dose and high-dose mitomycin trabeculectomy as an initial surgery in primary open-angle glaucoma. *Ophthalmology* 1993;**100**:1624–8.

Lloyd MA, Baerveldt G, Fellenbaum PS et al. Intermediate-term results of randomized clinical trial of the 350 versus 500 mm Baerveldt Implant. *Ophthalmology* 1994;**101**:1463–4.

Lois N, Wong D, Groenwald C. New surgical approach in the surgical management of psuedophakic malignant glaucoma. *Ophthalmology* 2001; **108**: 780–3.

Migdal C, Hitchings R. Control of chronic simple glaucoma with primary medical, surgery and laser treatment. *Trans Ophthalmol Soc UK* 1986;**105**:653–6.

Molteno ACB. New implant for drainage in glaucoma: clinical trial. *Br J Ophthalmol* 1979;**53**:606–15.

Quigley HA, Maumenee AE. Long-term follow-up of treated open-angle glaucoma. *Am J Ophthalmol* 1979;**111**:51.

Sherwood MB, Migdal CS, Hitchings RA et al. Initial treatment of glaucoma. Surgery or medications. *Surv Ophthalmol* 1993;**37**:293.

Starita RJ, Fellman RL, Spaeth GL et al. Short and long-term effects of postoperative corticosteroids on trabeculectomy. *Ophthalmology* 1985;**92**:938.

Stewart WC, Chorak RP, Hunt HH et al. Factors associated with visual loss in patients with advanced glaucomatous changes in the optic nerve head. *Am J Ophthalmol* 1993;**116**:176.

The Fluorouracil Filtering Surgery Study Group. Three-year follow-up of the Fluorouracil Filtering Surgery Study. *Am J Ophthalmol* 1993;**115**:82.

Walton DS. Glaucoma in infants and children. In: Nelson LB, Calhoun JH, Harley RD, eds. Pediatric Ophthalmology, 3rd edn. Philadelphia: WB Saunders Company, 1991.

Wolner B, Liebman JM, Sassani JW et al. Late bleb-related endophthalmitis after trabeculectomy with adjunctive 5-fluorouracil. *Ophthalmology* 1991;**98**:1053.

Yang KJ, Moster MR, Azuara-Blanco A et al. Mitomycin-C supplemented trabeculectomy, phacoemulsification, and foldable lens implantation. *J Cataract Refract Surg* 1997;**23**:565.

14. NON-PENETRATING GLAUCOMA SURGERY

Tarek Shaarawy and André Mermoud

The first suggestion of a disease associated with a rise in intraocular pressure (IOP), thus corresponding to what is now known as glaucoma, seems to occur in the Arabian writings of Shams-ad-Deen of Cairo, the 13th-century Egyptian ophthalmologist who described a 'headache of the pupil, an illness associated with pain in the eye, hemicrania and dullness of the humors, followed by dilatation of the pupil and cataract; if it becomes chronic, tenseness of the eye and blindness supervened'. Ever since, the mainstay of glaucoma therapy has remained a battle to lower IOP, medically or surgically.

Trabeculectomy has been the gold standard of glaucoma surgery ever since Sugar in 1961 and Cairns in 1968 suggested a shift away from the then common full-thickness glaucoma filtering procedures. The use of a superficial flap was of paramount importance in creating a resistance to aqueous outflow, lowering the incidence of postoperative hypotony as well as offering a protection against the catastrophic occurrence of endophthalmitis.

Over the years, evidence mounted to show that trabeculectomy is perhaps not the ideal surgery for glaucoma. Most surgeons prefer to delay surgery because of the potential vision-threatening complications of classical trabeculectomy, with or without antimetabolites. Complications include hypotony, hyphaema, flat anterior chamber, choroidal effusion or haemorrhage, surgery-induced cataract, and bleb failure.

Despite the tendency to delay surgery, trabeculectomy remains a very effective way of lowering IOP. Some authors hypothesize that if the safety margin of glaucoma surgery could be increased significantly without sacrificing efficacy, surgical intervention for glaucoma might be considered earlier.

Mikhail Leonidovich Krasnov of the former USSR paved the ground for non-penetrating filtering surgery in 1967, when he published his pioneering work on what he called sinusotomy. Several techniques have since evolved, probably the most popular of which are deep sclerectomy and viscocanalostomy.

Principles of non-penetrating filtering surgery

The main idea behind non-penetrating filtering surgery is to somehow surgically enhance the natural aqueous outflow channels, rather than create a new and possibly overly effective drainage site. The avoidance of penetration into the anterior chamber should allow the anterior segment to recover more quickly, with less risk of hypotony and its sequelae.

In primary and in most cases of secondary open-angle glaucoma, the main aqueous outflow resistance is thought to be located at the level of the juxta-canalicular trabeculum and the inner wall of Schlemm's canal. These two anatomical structures can be removed. This technique was first proposed by Zimmermann in 1984, and he used the term 'ab-externo trabeculectomy' to describe it.

Another way to increase the aqueous outflow in a patient with restricted posterior trabeculum outflow is to remove the corneal stroma behind the anterior trabeculum and Descemet's membrane. This has been called deep sclerectomy and was first described by Fyodorov and Kozlov in 1989. After deep sclerectomy, the main aqueous outflow occurs at the level of the anterior trabeculum and Descemet's membrane, the so-called trabeculo-Descemet's membrane (TDM).

In viscocanalostomy, described by Stegmannn in 1995, the aqueous filters through the TDM to the scleral space, as in deep sclerectomy, but it does not form a subconjunctival filtering bleb because the superficial scleral flap is tightly closed. From the scleral space, the aqueous reaches the Schlemm's canal ostia, which are surgically opened, and dilated with a viscoelastic substance.

Technique of non-penetrating glaucoma surgery

Deep sclerectomy

3–4 mL of a solution of bupivacaine 0.75%, xylocaine 4% and hyaluronidase 50U are usually sufficient for a successful local anesthesia. Topical and subconjunctival anesthesia are also possible and have been successful in selected cases.

A superior rectus muscle traction suture is placed and the eyeball is rotated to expose the site of the deep sclerotomy (DS) (usually the superior quadrant). To avoid superior rectus muscle bleeding, a superior intracorneal suture may be placed, not too near from the limbus so that anterior dissection of DS is not harmed.

The conjunctiva is opened either at the limbus or in the fornix. The limbal incision offers a better scleral exposition but needs a more careful closure, especially when antimetabolites are used.

The sclera is exposed and moderate hemostasis is performed. To allow the scleral dissection, all Tenon's capsule residue should be removed with a hockey stick. Sites with large aqueous drainage veins have to be avoided, to preserve as much as possible of the aqueous humor physiological outflow pathways.

A superficial scleral flap measuring 5 × 5 mm is dissected including 1/3 of the scleral thickness (about 300 μm). The initial incision is done with a No. 11

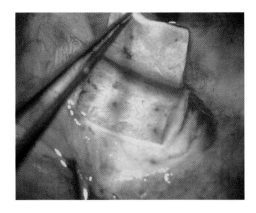

Figure 14.1 A superficial scleral flap measuring 5 × 5 mm is dissected including 1/3 of the scleral thickness (about 300 μm). In order to later be able to dissect the corneal stroma down to Descemet's membrane, the scleral flap is dissected 1–1.5 mm into clear cornea.

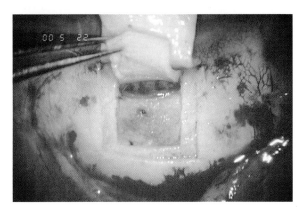

Figure 14.2 Deep sclero-keratectomy is done by performing a second deep scleral flap (4 × 4 mm). The deep flap is smaller than the superficial one leaving a step of sclera on the three sides. The remaining scleral layer should be as thin as possible (50–100 μm).

stainless steel blade. The horizontal dissection is done with a crescent ruby blade. In order to be able to dissect the corneal stroma down to Descemet's membrane, the scleral flap is dissected 1–1.5 mm into clear cornea. (Figure 14.1)

In patients with high risk of sclero-conjunctival scar formation (young, secondary glaucoma, and blacks), a sponge soaked in mitomycin-C 0.02% may be placed for 45 seconds in the scleral bed as well as between the sclera and the Tenon's capsule.

Deep sclero-keratectomy is done by making a second deep scleral flap (4 × 4 mm). The two lateral and the posterior deep scleral incisions are made using a 15-degree diamond blade. The deep flap is smaller than the superficial one leaving a step of sclera on the three sides (Figure 14.2). This will allow a tighter closure of the superficial flap in case of an intraoperative perforation of

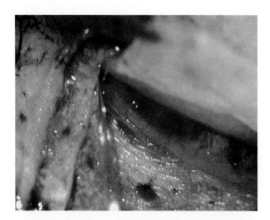

Figures 14.3 and 14.4
The inner wall of
Schlemm's canal and
juxtacanalicular trabeculum
are removed using a small
blunt forceps.

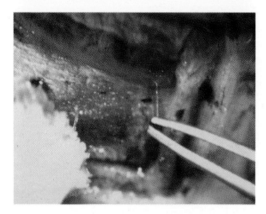

the TDM. The deep scleral flap is then dissected horizontally using the ruby blade. The remaining scleral layer should be as thin as possible (50–100 μm). Deep sclerectomy is preferably started in the posterior part of the deep scleral flap. Reaching the anterior part of the dissection, Schlemm's canal is unroofed. Schlemm's canal is located anterior to the scleral spur where the scleral fibers are regularly oriented, parallel to the limbus, however, in patients with congenital glaucoma, Schlemm's canal localization is more difficult, because it is often more posteriorly situated. Schlemm's canal is opened and the sclerocorneal dissection is prolonged anteriorly for 1–1.5 mm to remove the sclerocorneal tissue behind the anterior trabeculum and the Descemet's membrane. This step of the surgery is quite challenging because there is a high risk of perforation of the anterior chamber. The best way to perform this last dissection is to do two radial corneal cuts without touching the anterior trabeculum or the Descemet's membrane. This is performed with the 15-degree diamond knife (Figure 14.3). When the anterior dissection between corneal stroma and Descemet's membrane is completed, the deep scleral flap is cut anteriorly using the diamond knife. At this stage, there should be a diffuse percolation of aqueous through the remaining TDM.

The inner wall of Schlemm's canal and juxtacanalicular trabeculum are then removed using a small blunt forceps (Figure 14.4). The superficial scleral flap is then closed and secured with two loose 10/0 nylon sutures. So, in fact, the procedure has evolved into a combination of deep sclerectomy and ab-externo trabeculectomy.

The use of implants

To avoid a secondary collapse of the superficial flap over the TDM and the remaining scleral layer, a collagen implant is placed in the scleral bed and secured with a single 10/0 nylon suture (Figure 14.5). The implant is processed from porcine scleral collagen. It increases in volume after contact with aqueous and is slowly resorbed within 6 to 9 months, leaving a scleral space for aqueous filtration. Other implants may be used to fill the sclerocorneal space left after DS dissection: reticulated hyaluronic acid implant resorbing in about 3 months or T-shaped hydrophilic acrylic implant, which is non-absorbable. The role of implants in non-penetrating surgery is still controversial, but the bulk of studies comparing deep sclerectomy with an implant versus without, seem to show higher success rates with the use of an implant.

Viscocanalostomy

In viscocanalostomy, high-viscosity hyaluronic acid is injected into the two surgically created ostia of Schlemm's canal, aiming to dilate both the ostia and the canal. It is also placed in the scleral bed. The material is resorbed in 4–5 days.

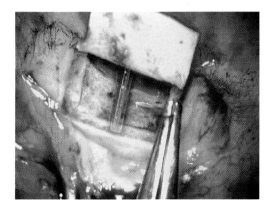

Figure 14.5 To avoid a secondary collapse of the superficial flap over the trabeculo-Descemet's membrane and the remaining scleral layer, a collagen implant is placed in the scleral bed and secured with a single 10/0 nylon suture.

The superficial scleral flap has to be tightly sutured to keep the viscoelastic substance in situ, and to force the aqueous to percolate through the TDM into the two ostia.

Nd-YAG goniopuncture after deep sclerectomy

When filtration through TDM is considered to be insufficient because of raised IOP, Nd:YAG goniopuncture should be performed. Using a gonioscopy contact lens, the aiming beam is focused on the semi-transparent TDM. Using the free running Q switched mode, with a power of 4–5 mJ, two to 15 shots are applied. This should result in the formation of microscopic holes through the TDM, allowing a direct passage of aqueous from the anterior chamber to the subconjunctival space. The success rate of Nd:YAG laser goniopuncture is satisfactory, with an immediate reduction in IOP of about 50%. The success of goniopuncture depends mainly on the thickness of the TDM, hence the importance of sufficiently deep intraoperative dissection.

By opening the TDM, however, goniopuncture transforms a non-perforating filtration procedure into a microperforating one. Some surgeons argue that since goniopuncture is done commonly after deep sclerectomy, the surgery is in fact a perforating procedure done in two stages (47% of deep sclerectomy patients in a long-term study had goniopunctures). The fact remains that prevention of perforation intraoperatively and in the early postoperative period seems to dramatically lower the incidence of complications. Although the potential risk of late bleb-related endophthalmitis may be increased after goniopuncture, no such cas has ever been reported.

Mechanism of filtration of non-penetrating filtering surgery

There are two sites of interest when discussing mechanism of filtration:

Flow through trabeculo-Descemet's membrane

The TDM offers sufficient resistance to aqueous outflow to ensure a slow decrease in IOP during surgery, and accounts for the reliable and reproducible IOP on the first postoperative day. Thus the main advantage of the TDM is in reducing the immediate postoperative complications. The main outflow through the TDM probably occurs at the level of the anterior trabeculum and not through the Descemet's membrane.

Aqueous humor resorption

Following aqueous percolation through the TDM, it is resorbed through:

Subconjunctival bleb

In almost all cases of deep sclerectomy, a diffuse, subconjunctival bleb is observed in the first postoperative day. Years after the operation, using ultrasonic biomicroscopy (UBM) assessment, all successful cases still showed a low profile diffused subconjunctival filtering bleb. This bleb, however, is usually smaller than the one seen after trabeculectomy.

Intrascleral bleb

When deep sclerectomy is performed a certain volume of sclera is removed, ranging between 5 and 8 mm^3. If the superficial scleral flap does not collapse, this scleral volume may be transformed into an intrascleral filtering bleb. UBM examination shows an intrascleral bleb in more than 90% of cases.

Subchoroidal space

Since the remaining layer of sclera after deep sclerectomy is very thin, there may be a drainage of aqueous humor into the suprachoroidal space. Using UBM, it is possible to observe fluid between the ciliary body and the remaining sclera in 45% of patients studied years after deep sclerectomy (unpublished data). Hypothetically, aqueous in the choroidal space may reach the uveoscleral outflow, and could also induce a chronic ciliary body detachment, thereby reducing aqueous production.

Schlemm's canal

On either side of a deep sclerectomy, the two ostia of Schlemm's canal may drain the aqueous humor into the episcleral veins. This mechanism may be more important after viscocanalostomy since the Schlemm's canal is dilated with high viscosity hyluronic acid.

Clinical results and advantages of non-penetrating filtering surgery

In a prospective non-randomized trial comparing 44 patients who had medically uncontrolled primary open-angle glaucoma and underwent deep sclerectomy with collagen implant (DSCI), with a matched group of 44 patients who underwent trabeculectomy, the complete success rate defined as an IOP lower than 21 mmHg without medication was 69% 24 months postoperatively in the deep sclerectomy group, versus 57% in the trabeculectomy group.

In another non-randomized prospective trial, 100 eyes of 100 consecutive patients with medically uncontrolled primary and secondary open-angle glaucoma underwent deep sclerectomy with collagen implant. Complete success rate, defined as an IOP lower than 21 mmHg without medication, was 44.6% at 36 months. Qualified success rate, defined as an IOP lower than 21 mmHg with and without medication, was 97.7% at 36 months. In a recent study, Shaarawy and colleagues reported that after 5 years, the mean IOP of 105 patients who underwent deep sclerectomy with collagen implant was 11.8 mmHg. Complete success rate was 63% and qualified success was 95.1%. Perhaps the real advantage of non-penetrating filtering surgery can be summarized in one sentence: DSCI may offer similar success rate to trabeculectomy, with fewer complications.

Conclusion

Non-penetrating filtering surgeries performed by several investigators offer a significant fall in IOP and satisfactory success rate after several years of follow-up for all types of open-angle glaucoma. The immediate postoperative complications are few, and visual acuity is almost unaffected. This is mainly due to the presence of the TDM, which allows a progressive drop in IOP and offers enough resistance to prevent immediate postoperative complications. When comparing trabeculectomy, the gold standard, with non-penetrating filtering surgery, the newcomer; it is perhaps wiser to remember the words of Heraclitus, uttered thousands of years ago: '*Nothing endures but change*'.

Suggested references for further reading

Mermoud A, Schnyder C, Sickenberg M et al. Comparison of deep sclerectomy with collagen implant and trabeculectomy in open angle glaucoma. *J Cataract Refract Surg* 1999;**25**:323–31.

Sanchez E, Schnyder CC, Sickenberg M et al. Deep sclerectomy: results with and without collagen implant. *Int Ophtalmol* 1997;**20**:157–62.

Shaarawy T, Karlen ME, Sanchez E et al. Long term results of deep sclerectomy with collagen implant. *Acta Ophthalmol Scand* 2000;**78**:323.

Stegmann RC. Viscocanalostomy: a new surgical technique for open angle glaucoma. *An Inst Barraquer, Spain* 1995;**25**:229–32.

15. TREATMENT OVERVIEW

Augusto Azuara-Blanco, Richard P Wilson, and Vital P Costa

Treatment goals

Many factors impact the quality of life of patients with glaucoma. These include the functional loss due to the disease, the anxiety and worry associated with the diagnosis of a chronic and potentially blinding disease, and the inconvenience, side-effects and cost of treatment.

The goal of glaucoma therapy is to prevent visual disability and to preserve the quality of life for the expected lifetime of the patient with minimal or no side-effects.

How should we treat glaucoma?

Lowering intraocular pressure (IOP) is currently the only option proven to be effective to slow or halt the deterioration of visual function in glaucoma. There is evidence that lowering IOP below 15 mmHg preserves the visual field in most patients with advanced primary open-angle glaucoma. The Advanced Glaucoma Intervention Study (AGIS) suggests that an IOP of 12 mmHg is the optimum to avoid further loss of visual field with an acceptable risk of side-effects. Therefore, our primary treatment is to lower IOP, by either medical or surgical means.

Other potential causative risk factors should be addressed if possible. In this regard, current clinical trials will assess the effect of blood flow modulation and neuroprotection in glaucoma patients. Nocturnal systemic hypotension is associated with progression of glaucoma. Avoiding the evening dose of a hypotensive drug may be advisable in patients with progressive glaucoma using systemic antihypertensive agents and topical β-blockers. In the long-term, genetic therapy may play a role in the management of different types of glaucoma.

When should we start treatment?

In practical terms, treatment should be started whenever glaucomatous damage is detected or when the degree of IOP increase or other risk factors are such that future damage is likely. In patients with ocular hypertension, a general rule is to start treatment when the IOP is in the high 20s in the absence of other risk factors. Relevant risk factors, such as family history of visual loss related to glaucoma, pseudoexfoliation, pigment dispersion, or systemic hypotension, to name a few, mandate treatment with IOPs in the mid 20s if the patient's expected lifespan justifies intervention.

However, the efficacy of pressure lowering in preventing the development of glaucoma in eyes with ocular hypertension is not clear. Should we treat patients with high IOPs (e.g. > 26 mmHg) without detectable optic nerve or visual field damage? If waiting represents minimal risk to a patient's visual function, then we could avoid the adverse effects of treatment. Two prospective, controlled studies, the Ocular Hypertension Treatment Study (OHTS) and the Early Manifest Glaucoma Trial, will try to answer the above questions.

How much treatment should we give? Target pressure

The fundamental question that arises every time antiglaucoma therapy is initiated is the degree to which the IOP should be lowered. Setting a target pressure is part science and part of the art of medicine. A 'target pressure' can be defined as the IOP expected to prevent further glaucomatous damage.

It is obviously difficult to determine in advance the IOP level at which further damage will not occur in each patient. The target IOP can be adjusted depending on the response to therapy and the anticipated iatrogenic risk of the next treatment or intervention.

Several important factors should be taken into account when establishing a target pressure:

Severity of damage

The main guide to clinical decisions in glaucoma is the degree of damage already present and its rate of progression. As a general rule, the greater the glaucoma damage to the optic nerve, the lower the IOP should be to prevent further loss. In eyes with advanced glaucoma with threatened fixation, the target pressure should be adjusted downward because there is little margin of error (frequently close to 10 mmHg). Conversely, 'overtreating' patients with high IOP and mild or no damage should be avoided. For example, in patients with ocular hypertension with an initial IOP in the 30s and no additional risk factors, a reasonable target IOP would be 24 mmHg.

Age and life expectancy of the patient

The longer the life expectancy of the patient, the more aggressive the therapy should be.

Susceptibility of the optic nerve to damage, pressure level before treatment, and type of glaucoma

For example, if only mild damage has occurred at a pressure in the 40s, then IOP reduction to the low 20s may be acceptable. In this situation, we may assume that the optic nerve is relatively resistant to high pressures. On the other hand, if the same amount of damage occurred as a result of pre-treatment pressures in the low 20s, then reduction of pressure to the low to mid-teens may be necessary, because the optic nerve is probably more susceptible to damage. As a general rule, the IOP should be lowered 25–30% from levels at which glaucoma damage was ongoing to stop progression, and up to 40% to gain the potential for a slight improvement in the visual field.

The main limitation of using target pressure is that we measure IOP infrequently, whereas an eye is subjected to the effect of IOP continuously, with marked variations from hour to hour and day to day. A recent study suggested that a patient with lower average IOP but marked variablity of IOP was more at risk than a patient with steady but higher average IOP.

General strategy to treat glaucoma

The following step-wise approach may be helpful when facing a patient with glaucoma:

1 Document the initial functional and structural status and estimate the degree of visual disability. This requires a complete ocular examination, disc drawing, visual fields, and disc photos and/or computerized optic nerve topography analysis.
2 Select a target IOP expected to halt further progression of the disease and maintain IOP at or below this target level.
3 Monitor and minimize the side-effects associated with treatment.
4 Educate and engage the patient in the management of the disease. Education and encouragement will enhance compliance and acceptance by the patient.
5 Monitor status of the optic disc, visual fields and visual disability.
6 Reset the target IOP to a lower level if deterioration occurs.

Medications are usually the first line of treatment. A monocular therapeutic trial, in which the untreated eye serves as a control during the trial period, will determine efficacy and acceptance by the patient.

Laser trabeculoplasty can be very effective in some patients with primary open angle glaucoma (elderly, with moderate or intense pigmentation of the trabecular meshwork), pigmentary glaucoma and pseudoexfoliative glaucoma.

255

Laser treatment may be considered as a primary option in some glaucoma patients. The Glaucoma Laser Trial and the Glaucoma Laser Trial Follow-up Study highlighted the benefits of laser trabeculoplasty as a safe and effective initial treatment for glaucoma in the select group above.

The Collaborative Initial Glaucoma Treatment Study compares filtering surgery with medical treatment in newly diagnosed POAG. Each arm is followed by laser trabeculoplasty if treatment is inadequate. Outcome parameters are visual field testing, visual acuity, and quality-of-life assessment based on a standardized questionnaire. This study will provide important information on the effect of varying treatment methods in patients with glaucoma.

The promising role of non-penetrating trabeculectomy (deep sclerectomy with collagen implant and viscocanalostomy) awaits further investigation and long-term follow-up. Trabeculectomy (guarded filtering procedure or GFP) is currently the surgical procedure of choice. Antifibrotic agents are used in high-risk cases, although some surgeons routinely use antifibrotic agents in all filtering procedures. If failure occurs, repeated GFP with mitomycin-C is recommended. The next surgical option to lower IOP and preserve visual function is the implantation of an aqueous shunt. Cyclodestructive procedures are usually the last line of intervention in recalcitrant glaucomas.

Compliance

Glaucoma is a chronic, symptom-free disease, which requires long-term, costly treatment. Glaucoma medications are all associated with side-effects, and usually result in no subjective improvement. For these reasons, it is not surprising that non-compliance is so common among glaucoma patients. At least one third of patients do not comply with health-care recommendations. In certain circumstances, this proportion can be higher. Most patients with chronic glaucoma have mild or no symptoms and the consequences of stopping therapy are delayed. As a result, at least one-third to two-thirds of patients use their medications suboptimally. Non-compliance has been estimated to account for 10% of visual loss from glaucoma, and is an important cause of glaucoma blindness.

Patients will often volunteer that they do not comply with a prescribed medical regimen. At the same time, they will freely admit that they are careful to take their drops before their visit to the ophthalmologist's office. When such patients can be clearly identified and their behavior cannot be corrected, laser or surgical intervention should be recommended. More troublesome are patients who default on their treatment but will not admit it. Ophthalmologists are commonly unable to distinguish patients with poor compliance and conclude that these patients are not responding to their medication or, if the patients only take their medication before their doctors' appointments, are showing progression of their glaucoma at normal IOPs. Either conclusion results in erroneous treatment.

Compliance is enhanced when patients are made fully aware of the nature of the glaucomatous process and the consequences of the lack of compliance, when the therapeutic regime is minimized and tailored to the patient's daily schedule, and when drop instillation technique is demonstrated and the patient's ability to administer their medication is observed in the office. Overbearing instructions such as 'You have to take your drops or you will go blind,' only increase anxiety and denial and may decrease compliance. Directing the compliance discussion to a patient's core concerns is much more effective. For example, 'I know your ability to drive keeps you from being dependent on your daughter for groceries and doctors' appointments. I'm afraid if we can't arrest your glaucoma damage, you may lose this ability.' Cooperating with primary-care physicians, minimizing side-effects, and improving the doctor-patient relationship will also improve a patient's compliance.

Suggested reading

Collaborative Normal Tension Glaucoma Study Group. Comparison of glaucomatous progression between untreated patients with normal-tension glaucoma and patients with therapeutically reduced intraocular pressures. *Am J Ophthalmol* 1998;**126**:487.

Collaborative Normal Tension Glaucoma Study Group. The effectiveness of intraocular pressure reduction in the treatment of normal-tension glaucoma. *Am J Ophthalmol* 1998;**126**:498.

Costa VP, Comegno PE, Vasconcelos JP et al. Low-dose mitomycin C trabeculectomy in patients with advanced glaucoma. *J Glaucoma* 1996;**5**:193–9.

Epstein DL, Krug Jr LH, Hertzmark E et al. A long-term clinical trial of timolol therapy versus no treatment in the management of glaucoma suspects. *Ophthalmology* 1989;**96**:1460.

Glaucoma Laser Trial Research Group. The Glaucoma Laser Trial (GLT) and Glaucoma Laser Trial Follow-up Study. 7. Results. *Am J Ophthalmol* 1995;**120**:718.

Grant WM, Burke J. Why do some people go blind from glaucoma? *Ophthalmology* 1982;**89**:991–8.

Kass MA, Gordon MO, Hoff MR et al. Topical timolol administration reduces the incidence of glaucomatous damage in ocular hypertensive individuals. A randomized, double-masked, long-term clinical trial. *Arch Ophthalmol* 1989;**107**:1590–8.

Katz J, Sommer A. Risk factors for primary open-angle glaucoma. *Am J Prev Med* 1988;**4**:110.

Lesk MR, Spaeth GL, Azuara-Blanco A et al. Reversal of optic disc cupping after glaucoma surgery analyzed with a scanning laser tomograph. *Ophthalmology* 1999;**106**:1013.

The Advanced Glaucoma Intervention Study (AGIS): 7. The relationship between control of intraocular pressure and visual field deterioration. *Am J Ophthalmol* 2000;**130**:429.

The Fluorouracil Filtering Surgery Study Group. Five-year follow-up of the Fluorouracil Filtering Surgery Study. *Am J Ophthalmol* 1996;**121**:349.

INDEX

Note: Page references in *italics* refer to figures; those in **bold** refer to tables

metipranolol 166, 167
microspherophakia 129, *130*
migraine 105
    as risk factor for glaucoma 103
mitomycin-C 209, 210, *210*, 225
mitotic drugs 161–2
Molteno implant 233
Morning Glory syndrome 52
mydriasis 166
myopia 52
    as risk factor for glaucoma 102
    as risk factor for retinal detachment 163

nanophthalmos 155–6
nasal cupping *52*, 53
nasal steps 75, *75*
Nd-YAG goniopuncture after deep
    sclerectomy 250
Nd:YAG laser ididectomy 116
Nd:YAG laser peripheral iridotomy 114, *114*
neovascular glaucoma 111, 130–3, *132*
neovascular membranes 36
neuron cell death 15
neuroretinal rim 13
non-contact tonometers 25
non-penetrating glaucoma surgery 245–57
    advantages 251–2
    clinical results 251–2
    filtration mechanism 250–1
        aqueous humor resorption 251
        flow through trabeculo-Descemet's
            membrane 250
    principles 245–6
    technique 246–9
    use of implants 249
normal-tension glaucoma (NTG) 27, 101,
    105–8
notching 50, 53, *54*

Octopus perimeter 76
ocular hypertension 26
ocular surgery, glaucomas associated with
    139–41
ocular trauma 45, 105, 123–5
Ocusert system 163, *163*
open-angle glaucomas 42–5
optic disc drusen 84
optic disc hemorrhage 56, *57*
optic disc *see* optic nerve head

optic nerve
    anatomy 10–14
    damage
        pathophysiology 14–15
        susceptibility to 255
    head, anatomy 12–14
    topography 62, *62*
optic nerve head
    anatomy 12–14, *12*
    arterial vascularization *13*, *14*
    asymmetry *51*, 51–2
    drawing 58–9
    examination and documentation 57–60
    glaucomatous changes 49–56
    normal 50, *50*
    photographs 59–60
    quantitative measurements 61–5
optic papilla *see* optic nerve head
optic pits 104
Optical Coherence Tomography (OCT) 64
orbital varices 134
overpass cupping 53, *55*
pallor
    development of 50
    of neuroretinal rim 53–4
panretinal photocoagulation 132–3
pars plana 3
pars plicata 3–4
parvocellular (P) ganglion cells 11
pattern standard deviation (PSD) 81
pediatric glaucoma 147–56
    differential diagnosis **148**
    incidence 147
    treatment 150–1
peripapillary atrophy 54–6, *56*
peripheral anterio synechiae 36
peripheral iris configuration 37
Perkins tonometer 25
Peters' anomaly 45, 153, *154*
phacoanaphylaxis 128
phacolytic glaucoma 126, *126*
phacomorphic glaucoma 128–9
phospholine iodide 164
photogrammetry 62
photophobia 147
PhXA34 172
pigment dispersion syndrome (PDS) 36, 42,
    44, 121, *122*
pigmentary glaucoma 121–3